St. Anthony's

# Clinical CODER

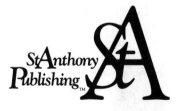

StAnthony
Publishing™

# Disclaimer

*St. Anthony's Clinical Coder* has been prepared based upon subjective medical judgment and upon the information available as of the date of publication. This publication is designed to provide accurate and authoritative information in regard to the subject covered, and every reasonable effort has been made to ensure the accuracy of the information contained within these pages. *St. Anthony's Clinical Coder* serves only as a guide. St. Anthony Publishing, Inc., its employees, agents and staff make no representation or guarantee that the use of this *Clinical Coder* will prevent differences or opinion or disputes with Medicare or other payers as to the amounts which will be paid to providers of services. St. Anthony Publishing, Inc., its employees, agents and staff make no representation or guarantee that this *Clinical Coder* is free of errors and will bear no responsibility or liability for the results or consequences of its use.

## *Acknowledgments*

The following staff contributed to the preparation of this book:

Marleeta K. Jones, *executive vice president, health care services*
Nancy Estler Grambo, *vice president, product development*
Connie Johnson, ART, CCS, *technical editor*
Karen Schmidt, BSN, *technical editor*
Lisa Woodward, *book production manager*
Keith L. Swann, MA, BA, *managing editor*
Regina Kukucka, *copy editor*
Marna Grim, *cover design*


Please address all correspondence to:

Director, Health Resources Group
St. Anthony Publishing, Inc.
11410 Isaac Newton Square
Reston, VA 20190
(800) 632-0123

ISBN 1-56329-347-1

# Table of Contents

# Introduction

Our experience shows that medical record reviewers often are forced to spend time and energy locating, obtaining and cross-referencing various resources that they need to do their jobs. Many times these resources are obsolete due to the frequent changes in medical practice and to new developments in scientific technology.

*St. Anthony's Clinical Coder* is a compilation of the most up-to-date resources available for reviewing medical records. The *Clinical Coder* assists health care professionals in defining and interpreting test results, laboratory values, drug usage and treatments. It also serves as a guide for the identification of complications and comorbid conditions (CCs), a useful tool for accurate coding and proper reimbursement.

The *Clinical Coder* is divided into seven easy-to-use sections: Abnormal EKGs, Abnormal Laboratory Values, Organisms, Drug Usage, Most Commonly Missed CC Conditions, Cardiovascular Complications and Complex Diagnoses.

- **Abnormal EKGs:** This section lists abnormalities that may appear on an electrocardiogram (EKG), drugs that may be used to treat each problem, signs and symptoms that may be present and possible conditions associated with the abnormality.

- **Abnormal Laboratory Values:** This section lists the batteries of laboratory tests by their specific test results, conditions indicated by the tests, signs and symptoms and common treatment modalities. A reference range of normal values is provided for each laboratory test. These values reflect test result differences that arise from the variety of laboratory equipment available. A space is provided to fill in the hospital's normal range for each laboratory test.

- **Organisms:** This is a handy reference that lists the organism growth normal to a particular body site. This information is listed, for each body site, under the heading "Normal Condition of Flora." A range of possible pathogens that may indicate an infectious process also is listed for each body site. The source and site of each specimen are identified for further clarification.

- **Drug Usage:** This is a quick alphabetic reference for commonly prescribed drugs, along with their generic names. Quick review of a patient's medication record may indicate a list of prescribed drugs for which a diagnosis is not listed. This section will help the coder locate the drug and determine the drug action and the indications for the drug.

- **Most Commonly Missed CC Conditions:**  This section lists CCs that the coder should look for in the medical record. The listing includes the signs and symptoms and ancillary report findings that indicate the presence of particular CCs.

- **Cardiovascular Complications:**  This section provides a comprehensive list of the recognized cardiovascular complications that affect diagnosis-related group (DRG) 121, circulatory disorders with acute myocardial infarction and cardiovascular complication, discharged alive. Signs and symptoms and ancillary report findings that indicate complications also are listed.

- **Complex Diagnoses:**  This section includes the diagnoses that affect DRG 124, circulatory disorders (except acute myocardial infarction) with cardiac catheterization and complex diagnosis. The list contains complex diagnoses, their signs and symptoms and the ancillary report findings that indicate the presence of certain conditions. Note that the italicized diagnosis codes in brackets are manifestation codes, which represent underlying conditions, and should not be used to describe principal diagnosis.

# General Instructions

*St. Anthony's Clinical Coder* is used by a variety of health care professionals—utilization review and quality assurance coordinators, peer review organization (PRO) reviewers, DRG coordinators, third-party payer reviewers and medical record coders. It also serves as a quick reference in hospital, physician or freestanding laboratories.

The *Clinical Coder* assists health care professionals in determining whether potentially overlooked conditions can be coded. Accurate code assignment depends on the record reviewer looking for the following two items:

1.  Abnormal test results
2.  Documentation of treatment (such as medication) for an abnormality.

***Example:***
A patient's principal diagnosis is pneumonia. The specific cause of the pneumonia is not indicated in the medical record, although certain kinds of pneumonia may increase the resources used to treat a patient.

Turn in the *Clinical Coder* to the Organisms section, arranged by site of specimen. Note from the laboratory findings in the medical record that a sputum culture grew *S. aureus.* Look under "Sputum," the specimen source, in the Organisms section. Notice that *S. aureus* is pathogenic in this instance. After verification with the physician that *S. aureus* is the causative organism of the patient's pneumonia, the physician modifies the principal diagnosis to read "pneumonia due to *S. aureus.*"

Next, determine whether there are any secondary diagnoses, as they could mean that additional resources were used to treat the patient. Although the physician has not stated any secondary diagnoses in this case, a review of the medical record—especially ancillary reports—may suggest additional diagnoses or conditions.

In this example, compare the patient's laboratory test results with the results listed in the Abnormal Laboratory Values section of the *Clinical Coder.* This section lists various abnormal test results, the possible conditions they indicate, along with the signs, symptoms and treatment of those conditions. If the test results fall outside of the hospital's reference range for the test, which is indicated in the upper right-hand corner of each page in the section, the patient could have one of the conditions listed beneath the test.

Remember, the medical record must include documentation (physician progress notes, ancillary report findings) that confirms the presence of the condition. Clinical evidence must support principal and subsequent diagnoses before they can be reported.

In this instance, investigating the laboratory values reveals that the patient had a urine culture that showed an *E. coli* colony growth of greater than 100,000. According to the Abnormal Laboratory Values section, under "Urine Culture—Presence of Pathogens," this abnormal finding indicates the possible presence of a urinary tract infection.

To determine whether a 100,000 colony count of *E. coli* is significant in this instance, look under "Urine" in the Organisms section. The information under "Possible Pathogens" lists any organism with a count greater than 100,000 as infectious.

Next, check the medication record for evidence that the patient was treated for a urinary tract infection. For this example, the physician prescribed Septra. Look up "Septra" in the Drug Usage section of the *Clinical Coder*. Note that the medication frequently is used to treat urinary tract infections.

This example shows that the coder can detect evidence of a urinary tract infection by reviewing the patient's medical record, along with referencing the appropriate sections in the *Clinical Coder*. The evidence includes the abnormal results of the patient's urine culture and the medication record, which indicates that Septra was prescribed during the patient's hospital stay.

The next step is to ask the physician to add the omitted condition to the medical record, based on the clinical findings and treatment documented in the record. For appropriate reimbursement, it is important to include the additional diagnosis code to complete the patient's profile.

# Chapter 1:  Abnormal EKGs

| Abnormal Tracing | Documentation |
|---|---|
| **Arrhythmias** | • *Condition:*  Atrioventricular (AV) block, third-degree; sometimes called complete heart block with (possible) angina pectoris<br><br>*Signs and Symptoms:*  Dizziness, syncope, dyspnea<br><br>*Drugs:*   Treatment is insertion of a pacemaker; however, drugs like atropine, epinephrine and isoproterenol may be used temporarily until a pacemaker is placed<br><br>• *Condition:*  Trifascicular block<br><br>*Signs and Symptoms:*  Dizziness, syncope, dyspnea<br><br>*Drugs:*   Treatment is insertion of a pacemaker, however drugs like atropine, epinephrine and isoproterenol may be used temporarily until a pacemaker is placed |
| **Arrhythmias, atrial premature ventricular contractions (PVCs), right bundle branch block, p-pulmonale, right axis deviation** | • *Condition:*   Cor pulmonale is a term applied to enlargement of the right ventricle resulting from pulmonary hypertension, most often due to chronic obstructive pulmonary disease (COPD).<br><br>Patients usually exhibit a long course of slowly deteriorating exercise tolerance due to shortness of breath and edema.<br><br>Sudden decompensation is known as acute cor pulmonale and is most often due to a massive pulmonary embolus.<br><br>*Drugs:*  Bronchodilators, steroids, diuretics, digitalis, antibiotics.  Occasionally heparin or Tissue Plasminogen Activator (TPA) are given if pulmonary embolus is present. |
| **Arrhythmias of all types due to electrolyte imbalance** | • *Condition:*  Acute renal failure<br><br>*Signs and Symptoms:*  Lethargy, fatigue, anorexia, nausea, dyspnea, weakness, thirst, oliguria, bradycardia or tachycardia; can develop as a complication of congestive heart failure, shock or sepsis<br><br>*Drugs:*  Type of arrhythmia dictates specific drug prescribed |

| Abnormal Tracing | Documentation |
|---|---|
| **Arrhythmias; S-T segment changes, cardiac monitoring usually necessary** | • *Condition:* Intermediate coronary syndrome<br><br>*Signs and Symptoms:* Anginal pain, history of chronic coronary insufficiency, possible exacerbation of previously stable angina; "pending infarction" also may be called "preinfarction syndrome"<br><br>*Drugs:* Varies per physician discretion |
| **Beats, premature atrial, abnormally shaped P waves, regular rhythm at 150-220 beats per minute** | • *Condition:* Paroxysmal supraventricular tachycardia<br><br>*Signs and Symptoms:* Abrupt onset and termination of palpitations; often asymptomatic, although patient may be aware of rapid heartbeat; some patients complain of throbbing vessels of the throat, dyspnea, sweating, dizziness, syncope, weakness, polyuria<br><br>*Drugs:* Digoxin, inderal, metoprolol, esmolol, verapamil, diltiazem, adenocard, quinidine, procainamide, norpace, soltolol, or mexiletine. |
| **Beats, uninterrupted series** | • *Condition:* Paroxysmal tachycardia<br><br>*Signs and Symptoms:* Fluttering sensation in chest, weakness, faintness, nausea<br><br>*Drugs:* May include quinidine, procainamide, tambocor or disopyramide |
| **Bradycardia (shown in changes prior to arrest), tachycardia or other arrhythmias, fibrillation or asystole** | • *Condition:* Cardiac arrest<br><br>*Signs and Symptoms:* Sudden unexpected cessation of cardiac action, absence of heart sounds and/or blood pressure; cardiopulmonary resuscitation (CPR) performed<br><br>*Drugs:* May include isoproterenol, atropine, sodium bicarbonate, epinephrine and calcium gluconate |

| Abnormal Tracing | Documentation |
|---|---|
| **Changes, junction J, S-T, T interval, T-U segment and U wave** | • *Condition:* Rupture of papillary muscle<br><br>*Signs and Symptoms:* Contraction of papillary muscle, possible chest pain and hemoptysis; deterioration usually sudden and severe; often manifestation of congestive heart failure with cyanosis and sometimes shock<br><br>*Drugs:* May include lasix or diuril |
| **Changes, S-T segment, inversion or flattening of T waves** | • *Condition:* Ischemia<br><br>*Signs and Symptoms:* Arteriosclerotic heart disease, elevated cholesterol disease of aortic valve, thoracic pain, anemia, dizziness, syncope, dyspnea, angina, palpation, neck or jaw pain or diaphoresis<br><br>*Drugs:* Nitroglycerin, oxygen, Beta-blockers, calcium channel blockers, vasodilators |
| **Complexes, QRS, chaotic and rapid ventricular rhythm** | • *Condition:* Ventricular fibrillation<br><br>*Signs and Symptoms:* Absence of effective cardiac action resulting in loss of pulse, respiration and blood pressure; a life-threatening cardiac emergency—seizures and death can occur<br><br>*Drugs:* Lidocaine, procainamide, bretylium tosylate, epinephrine |
| **Complex, QRS, lasting 0.12 seconds or longer, T wave essentially normal in all leads except V1-V3, left anterior fascicular block** | • *Condition:* Right bundle branch block and left anterior fascicular block<br><br>*Signs and Symptoms:* Usually asymptomatic<br><br>*Drugs:* Varies per physician discretion |

| Abnormal Tracing | Documentation |
|---|---|
| **Complexes, QRS, wide** | • *Condition:*  Paroxysmal ventricular tachycardia<br><br>*Signs and Symptoms:*  Associated with ischemic heart disease, especially myocardial infarction (MI); precordial pain, sudden onset usually preceded by premature ventricular beats, pulse rate of 150-210 beats per minute<br><br>*Drugs:*  May include antiarrhythmic medication (e.g., lidocaine, pronestyl) |
| **Contractions, premature atrial** | • *Condition:*  Functional disturbances following cardiac surgery<br><br>*Signs and Symptoms:*  History of cardiac surgery (may have occurred previously or during the present admission); functional disturbances may be indicated by arrhythmias, level of consciousness, diaphoresis or drop in blood pressure (diastolic pressure less than 60)<br><br>*Drugs:*  May include quinidine, lidocaine or pronestyl |
| **Deviation, axis features of right or left ventricular failure, hypertrophy** | • *Condition:*  Rupture of chordae tendonae<br><br>*Signs and Symptoms:*  Usually sudden in onset with chest pain, possibly dyspnea and weakness; caused by bacterial endocarditis, trauma or sudden compression of thorax<br><br>*Drugs:*  May include use of diuretics for congestive heart failure (e.g., lasix) |
| **Deviation, S-T segment, bradycardia, tachycardia, fibrillation or asystole** | • *Condition:*  Cardiac arrest<br><br>*Signs and Symptoms:*  Sudden cessation of cardiac action, absence of heart sounds or blood pressure<br><br>*Drugs:*  Isoproterenol, atropine, sodium bicarbonate, epinephrine, lidocaine |

| Abnormal Tracing | Documentation |
|---|---|
| **Disassocia-tion, AV, sudden onset; block may be 2 to 1, 3 to 1, or 4 to 1** | • *Condition:* Atrioventricular block, Mobitz type II; also called partial or incomplete heart block<br><br>*Signs and Symptoms:* Attack of syncope related to sudden cessation of circulation in upright or recumbent position<br><br>*Drugs:* Atropine for bradycardia; discontinuation of digitalis |
| **Elevation, S-T segment T wave changes, bundle branch abnor-mality** | • *Condition:* Aneurysm of heart wall<br><br>*Signs and Symptoms:* Palpitations, severe dyspnea, generalized edema (may occur after an MI)<br><br>*Drugs:* Varies per physician discretion |
| **Fibrillation, atrial** | • *Condition:* Functional disturbances following cardiac surgery<br><br>*Signs and Symptoms:* History of cardiac surgery (may have occurred previously or during the present admission); functional disturbances may be indicated by arrhythmias, level of consciousness, diaphoresis or drop in blood pressure (diastolic pressure less than 60)<br><br>*Drugs:* May include quinidine, lidocaine or Pronestyl<br><br>• *Condition:* Hypertensive and arteriosclerotic heart disease, myocardial infarction<br><br>Signs and Symptoms: Palpitations, near-syncope, pallor, nausea, weakness, lightheadedness and fatigue.<br><br>*Drugs:* Digitalis, quinidine sulfate, procainamide, verapamil |

| Abnormal Tracing | Documentation |
|---|---|
| **Fibrillation, ventricular** | • *Condition:* Cardiogenic shock<br><br>*Signs and Symptoms:* Hypotensive with poor perfusion usually results from massive myocardial infarction leading to severe left ventricular dysfunction, hypotension, pulmonary edema. Prognosis is very poor with mortality rate of >50%.<br><br>*Drugs:* Epinephrine, norepinephrine, dopamine, isoproterenol<br><br>• *Condition:* Functional disturbances following cardiac surgery<br><br>*Signs and Symptoms:* History of cardiac surgery (may have occurred previously or during the present admission); functional disturbances may be indicated by arrhythmias, level of consciousness, diaphoresis or drop in blood pressure (diastolic pressure less than 60)<br><br>*Drugs:* May include quinidine, lidocaine or pronestyl |
| **Fibrillation, ventricular and/or conduction defect** | • *Condition:* Hypovolemic or septic shock<br><br>*Signs and Symptoms:* Septic shock due to management of underlying disease; onset of abrupt chills, nausea, vomiting, diarrhea; extreme exhaustion (prostration), hypotension, fever, chills<br><br>*Drugs:* IV antibiotics |

| Abnormal Tracing | Documentation |
|---|---|
| **Flutter, atrial** | • *Condition:* Functional disturbances following cardiac surgery<br><br>*Signs and Symptoms:* History of cardiac surgery (may have occurred previously or during the present admission); functional disturbances may be indicated by arrhythmias, level of consciousness, diaphoresis or drop in blood pressure (diastolic pressure less than 60)<br><br>*Drugs:* May include quinidine, lidocaine or pronestyl<br><br>• *Condition:* infarction, rheumatic heart disease<br><br>*Signs and Symptoms:* Atrial rate between 240 and 400%; palpitations, near-syncope, pallor, nausea, weakness, lightheadedness and fatigue<br><br>*Drugs:* Digitalis, quinidine sulfate, procainamide, verapamil |
| **Flutter, ventricular, regular rapid rate over 250 beats per minute** | • *Condition:* Ventricular flutter<br><br>*Signs and Symptoms:* Palpitations, dyspnea; possibly a transition between ventricular tachycardia and fibrillation<br><br>*Drugs:* Lidocaine, procainamide, bretylium |
| **Hypertrophy, left ventricular** | • *Condition:* Endocardial fibroelastosis<br><br>*Signs and Symptoms:* Cardiac hypertrophy with documentation of peripheral edema; usually occurs in ages six weeks to six months; in older children, there are usually poor heart sounds and often tachycardia; in patients over 50, history of six to 15 years of heart disease; possible relationship to mumps virus<br><br>*Drugs:* May include diuretics or digoxin |

| Abnormal Tracing | Documentation |
|---|---|
| **Infarction, myocardial, acute, PVCs, ventricular tachycardia** | • *Condition:* Shock<br><br>*Signs and Symptoms:* Hypotensive with poor perfusion usually results from massive myocardial infarction leading to severe left ventricular dysfunction, hypotension, pulmonary edema. Prognosis is very poor with mortality rate of >50%.<br><br>*Drugs:* Epinephrine, norepinephrine, dopamine, isoproterenol<br><br>• *Condition:* Postmyocardial infarction syndrome, called "Dressler syndrome"<br><br>*Signs and Symptoms:* Chest pain usually sharp and stabbing as that caused by infarction; aggravated by change in position and deep inspirations; usually follows an acute infarction by two to 11 weeks (appears to be like pleural effusion, pneumonitis with fever); pericardial friction rub present on auscultation |
| **P waves in regular rhythm (250 to 350 per minute), prolonged P-R interval, varying with degree of AV block** | • *Condition:* Atrial flutter<br><br>*Signs and Symptoms:* Palpitations, dyspnea, apprehension, dizziness, fainting; result of other conditions, such as acute myocardial infarction, angina, congestive heart failure and sepsis, or after bypass surgery<br><br>*Drugs:* Digoxin, inderal, metoprolol, esmolol, verapamil, diltiazem, adenocard, quinidine, procainamide, norpace, soltolol, or mexiletine |
| **Patterns producing an irregularly dropped beat that can be determined by cardiac auscultation or palpation of the pulse** | • *Condition:* Atrioventricular block<br><br>*Signs and Symptoms:* Dizziness, syncope, dyspnea<br><br>*Drugs:* Treatment is insertion of a pacemaker; however, drugs like atropine, epinephrine and isoproterenol may be used temporarily until a pacemaker is placed |

| Abnormal Tracing | Documentation |
|---|---|
| **QRS > 0.14 seconds with R-R1 in the leads V$_1$ + $_2$ and V$_5$ + $_6$** | • *Condition:* Bilateral bundle branch block<br><br>*Signs and Symptoms:* Usually asymptomatic<br><br>*Drugs:* No specific therapy |
| **QRS > 0.14 seconds with R-R1 morphology in the lateral lead of electrocardiogram (ECG)** | • *Condition:* Left bundle branch block<br><br>*Signs and Symptoms:* Usually asymptomatic; can be secondary to coronary artery disease or hypertension; makes the diagnosis of acute myocardial infarction more difficult<br><br>*Drugs:* No specific therapy |
| **Rate, atrial more than 400 beats per minute with a variable ventricular rate; P waves absent** | • *Condition:* Atrial fibrillation<br><br>*Signs and Symptoms:* Palpitations, dyspnea, apprehension, dizziness, fainting; result of other conditions, such as acute myocardial infarction, angina, congestive heart failure and sepsis, or after bypass surgery<br><br>*Drugs:* Digoxin, inderal, metoprolol, esmolol, verapamil, diltiazem, adenocard, quinidine, procainamide, norpace, soltolol, or mexiletine. |
| **Rhythm, ventricular, irregular regular atrial rhythm; often called "Wenckebach" pause** | • *Condition:* Atrioventricular, block, Mobitz I, second degree; also called partial or incomplete heart block<br><br>*Signs and Symptoms:* Weakness, faintness, palpitations, dyspnea, transient when in upright position; usually transient in nature and requires no treatment<br><br>*Drugs:* Atropine for bradycardia |
| **S-T, T wave abnormal** | • *Condition:* Aneurysm of coronary vessels<br><br>*Signs and Symptoms:* Palpitations, severe dyspnea, heart murmur, generalized edema<br><br>*Drugs:* Varies per physician discretion |

| Abnormal Tracing | Documentation |
|---|---|
| **T waves, low to inverted in most leads** | • *Condition:* Acute pericarditis in diseases classified elsewhere<br><br>*Signs and Symptoms:* Often a history of recent respiratory infection; precordial pain made worse by change of position, swallowing, coughing and deep breathing; dyspnea, chills, malaise are usually present; onset is sudden; the underlying condition (e.g., tuberculosis) also must be treated<br><br>• *Condition:* Acute pericarditis<br><br>*Signs and Symptoms:* Onset is usually abrupt and often preceded by sharp precordial or substernal pain radiating to the neck (precordial pain is distinguished from ischemic coronary pain because it usually is not aggravated by thoracic motion); fever, chills, weakness are common<br><br>• *Condition:* Hemopericardium<br><br>*Signs and Symptoms:* Results from a perforating trauma or cardiac rupture after myocardial infarction; symptoms include precordial pain, substernal oppression, dyspnea; death can result if emergency measures are not taken immediately<br><br>*Drugs:* As required to resuscitate patient |

| Abnormal Tracing | Documentation |
|---|---|
| **Tachycardia, atrial enlargement** | • *Condition:* Congestive heart failure<br><br>*Signs and Symptoms:* Dyspnea present with orthopnea and paroxysmal nocturnal dyspnea in more advanced failure; other symptoms include peripheral edema, irritability, weakness, sometimes cyanosis, irregular heart rate, moist rales in base of lungs with productive cough, confusion (usually present)<br><br>*Drugs:* Digoxin, diuretics, vasodilators<br><br>• *Condition:* Left heart failure<br><br>*Signs and Symptoms:* Hypertension, fatigue, cough, frothy sputum, pulmonary edema, dyspnea; possible cyanosis<br><br>*Drugs:* Diuretics, digoxin, vasodilators, dobutamine, amrinone<br><br>• *Condition:* Heart failure<br><br>*Signs and Symptoms:* Hypertension, fatigue, cough, frothy sputum, pulmonary edema, dyspnea; possible cyanosis<br><br>*Drugs:* Diuretics, digoxin, vasodilators, dobutamine, amrinone |
| **Tachycardia, bradycardia or PVCs** | • *Condition:* Hypertensive heart disease (benign) with congestive heart failure<br><br>*Signs and Symptoms:* Hypertension, fatigue, cough, frothy sputum, pulmonary edema, dyspnea; possible cyanosis<br><br>*Drugs:* Diuretics, digoxin, vasodilators, dobutamine, amrinone<br><br>• *Condition:* Hypertensive heart disease (malignant) with congestive heart failure<br><br>*Signs and Symptoms:* Hypertension, fatigue, cough, frothy sputum, pulmonary edema, dyspnea; confusion is usually present; possible cyanosis<br><br>*Drugs:* Diuretics, digoxin, vasodilators, dobutamine, amrinone |

| Abnormal Tracing | Documentation |
|---|---|
| **Tachycardia, intraventricular or bundle branch abnormalities, S-T segment changes, ventricular arrhythmias** | • *Condition:* Myocarditis, acute in diseases classified elsewhere<br><br>*Signs and Symptoms:* Associated with acute pericarditis, influenza, tuberculosis; precordial substernal discomfort, severe dyspnea, pain in right upper quadrant of abdomen<br><br>*Drugs:* May include antiarrhythmic drugs to control arrhythmias, antibiotics for underlying infection and antiinflammatory drugs<br><br>• *Condition:* Acute myocarditis<br><br>*Signs and Symptoms:* Usually persistent fever, fatigue, dyspnea, palpitations, chest discomfort, neck vein distention in the presence of accompanying congestive heart failure; rapidly progressive clinical course can be complicated by congestive heart failure<br><br>*Drugs:* May include antiarrhythmic drugs to control arrhythmias, antibiotics for underlying infection and antiinflammatory drugs<br><br>• *Condition:* Acute myocarditis; may be termed "interstitial"<br><br>*Signs and Symptoms:* Precordia, substernal discomfort, dyspnea, pain, fever; predominant physical findings are friction rub, leukocytosis, rapid sedimentation; there also may be evidence of generalized edema and/or ascites<br><br>*Drugs:* May include antiarrhythmic drugs to control arrhythmias, antibiotics for underlying infection and antiinflammatory drugs |

*continued*

| Abnormal Tracing | Documentation |
|---|---|
| **Tachycardia, intraventricular or bundle branch abnormalities, S-T segment changes, ventricular arrhythmias** *(continued)* | • *Condition:* Idiopathic myocarditis<br><br>*Signs and Symptoms:* MI, acute, possibly viral and parasitic infections, chills, weakness, discomfort in chest (precordial or substernal), onset of persistent fever<br><br>*Drugs:* May include antiarrhythmic drugs to control arrhythmias, antibiotics for underlying infection and antiinflammatory drugs<br><br>• *Condition:* Septic myocarditis<br><br>*Signs and Symptoms:* Viral strains, influenza viruses, bacteria<br><br>*Drugs:* May include antiarrhythmic drugs to control arrhythmias, antibiotics for underlying infection and antiinflammatory drugs<br><br>• *Condition:* Toxic myocarditis<br><br>*Signs and Symptoms:* May be caused by chemical poisons such as arsenic, excessive doses of drugs, excessive radiation exposure<br><br>*Drugs:* May include antiarrhythmic drugs to control arrhythmias, antibiotics for underlying infection and antiinflammatory drugs |
| **Tachycardia, PVCs, ventricular hypertrophy** | • *Condition:* Heart failure, left side<br><br>*Signs and Symptoms:* Hypertension, fatigue, cough, frothy sputum, pulmonary edema, dyspnea; confusion is usually present; possible cyanosis<br><br>*Drugs:* Diuretics, digoxin, vasodilators, dobutamine, amrinone |

| Abnormal Tracing | Documentation |
|---|---|
| **Tachycardia, S-T segment elevation, atrial arrhythmias** | • *Condition:* Idiopathic acute pericarditis<br><br>*Signs and Symptoms:* Precordial pain intensified by change in position, swallowing, coughing and deep breathing; dyspnea, chills, malaise and anorexia; onset is sudden in all ages; physical findings show pericardial friction rub; fever is usually greater than 102°<br><br>*Drugs:* IV antibiotics corticosteroids, antiinflammatory drugs such as aspirin and indocin |
| **Tachycardia, sinus** | • *Condition:* Hyperkinetic heart disease<br><br>*Signs and Symptoms:* Features of congestive heart failure such as cardiac enlargement, gallop rhythm, tachycardia; pulse pressure may be elevated (the difference between diastolic and systolic blood pressure is greater than 100)<br><br>*Drugs:* All types of antiangina medications and hypertensive drugs are possibilities |

| Abnormal Tracing | Documentation |
|---|---|
| **Tachycardia, sinus, all forms of heart block (i.e., first, second and third degree), junctional tachycardias** | • *Condition:* Infectious endocarditis, both acute and subacute, is due to infection of the lining of the heart manifested by development of fever, heart murmurs and persistent bacteremia. Collections of bacteria and inflammatory cells known as vegetations form on the heart lining and heart valves. Pieces of vegetations break loose and embolize to various organs (i.e., kidneys, nailbeds, lungs, etc.) causing damage to these organs and sometimes infection in these organs. |
| | Acute endocarditis is a clinical picture as described above accompanied by rapid destruction of heart valves with rapid deterioration of valve function leading to hemodynamic instability and heart failure. It is most often caused by Staphylococcus aureus infection of the heart. Its rapid progression is a result of the virulence of the Staphylococcus aureus organism. |
| | Subacute endocarditis represents a partially compensated form of infectious endocarditis, in which hemodynamic deterioration occurs very slowly, often over a period of weeks or months. It is most often due to infection with Streptococcus viridans, which is a much less virulent (or destructive) organism. |
| | *Drugs:* IV antibiotics |

| Abnormal Tracing | Documentation |
|---|---|
| **Tachycardia, sinus, atrial enlargement, PVCs, atrial fibrillation or ventricular hypertrophy** | • *Condition:* Primary cardiomyopathy<br><br>*Signs and Symptoms:* Usually occurs in elderly patients; evidenced by loss of consciousness, palpitations and/or dyspnea (palpitations may be indicated by bounding or rapid pulse, skipped heartbeats); edema and paroxysmal nocturnal dyspnea may be present; may include congestive and restrictive cardiomyopathies<br><br>*Drugs:* Antianginal medications, antihypertensives, presser agents, digoxin, diuretics<br><br>• *Condition:* Secondary cardiomyopathy<br><br>*Signs and Symptoms:* Dyspnea, paroxysmal nocturnal dyspnea, fatigue, edema, palpitations, hypertrophy of heart; occurs as a complication of cardiovascular disease or other systemic disease<br><br>*Drugs:* Digoxin, pronestyl, diuretics and vasodilators<br><br>• *Condition:* Alcoholic cardiomyopathy<br><br>*Signs and Symptoms:* Excessive alcohol intake, exertional dyspnea, cough, fatigue, hemoptysis and edema; frequently found in patients between the ages of 23 and 50<br><br>• *Condition:* Nutritional and metabolic cardiomyopathy<br><br>*Signs and Symptoms:* Dyspnea, paroxysmal nocturnal dyspnea, fatigue, edema, palpitations, high output heart failure; underlying disease is thyrotoxicosis, beriberi, amyloidosis<br><br>*Signs and Symptoms:* Increase in diastolic blood pressure, loss of consciousness, hypertrophy of heart and/or history of heart disease, dyspnea, paroxysmal nocturnal dyspnea, fatigue, edema, palpitations<br><br>• *Condition:* Cardiomyopathy in other diseases classified elsewhere |

| Abnormal Tracing | Documentation |
|---|---|
| **Tachycardia, "strain" patterns, LVH** | • *Condition:* Hypertensive heart and renal disease, malignant<br><br>*Signs and Symptoms:* History of renal disease, headache, fatigue, irritability, evidence of renal failure, elevated blood pressure (systolic greater than 160 and diastolic greater than 100), confusion may be present<br><br>*Drugs:* Nipride, vasodilators, nitroglycerin, B-blockers, procardia |
| **Tachycardia, ventricular, atrial flutter, supraventricular tachycardia (SVT)** | • *Condition:* Functional disturbances following cardiac surgery<br><br>*Signs and Symptoms:* History of cardiac surgery (may have occurred previously or during the present admission); functional disturbances may be indicated by arrhythmias, level of consciousness, diaphoresis or drop in blood pressure (diastolic pressure less than 60)<br><br>*Drugs:* May include quinidine, lidocaine or pronestyl |

# Chapter 2: Abnormal Laboratory Values

## Acetones or Ketones—
## Blood—Increased Level

**Reference Range: 0.3-2.0 Negative (A)**
**2-4 Negative (K)**

**Hospital Range:** _____

| Condition | Signs & Symptoms | Treatment |
|---|---|---|
| Ketoacidosis[§] | Excessive thirst, poly-uria, irritability, weakness | Restricted diet, monitoring of blood sugar levels |
| Ketosis, alco-holic[§] | Vomiting and dehydra-tion in association with other symptoms of alco-holism such as delirium tremens and cirrhosis | Intravenous infusion of normal saline and glucose |

[§] Complication or comorbid condition

# Acid Phosphatase—
# Blood—Increased Level

**Reference Range: 0.1-0.9**

**Hospital Range:** _____

| Condition | Signs & Symptoms | Treatment |
|---|---|---|
| **Cancer of prostate** | Urinary retention, urinary tract infections, palpable lesion of prostate. Bone pain is present with metastatic disease. | Surgery, hormone therapy, radiation therapy and chemotherapy may all be employed depending on the stage of the disease. |
| **Cirrhosis of liver**[§] | Abdominal pain or distention, fever, ascites, jaundice, anorexia | Sodium-restricted diet, intravenous fluids, treatment for relief of symptoms |
| **Failure, renal, chronic**[§] | Bruising, dyspnea, lethargy, weakness, anorexia, polyuria | Fluid restrictions, dialysis, transfusion(s) of blood and blood components |

[§] Complication or comorbid condition

# Albumin—
# Blood—Decreased Level

**Reference Range: 0.1-0.9**

**Hospital Range:** _____

| Condition | Signs & Symptoms | Treatment |
|---|---|---|
| **Burns** | Can result from thermal, electrical or chemical injuries. Severity is estimated by the size and depth of the burn. | Reverse isolation, skin grafts, intravenous fluids, invasive monitoring, high protein/high calorie diet |
| **Cirrhosis of liver**[§] | Abdominal pain or distention, fever, ascites, jaundice, anorexia | Sodium-restricted diet, intravenous fluids, treatment for relief of symptoms |
| **Syndrome, nephrotic**[§] | Edema, lethargy, anorexia, orthostatic hypotension | Diuretics, steroid therapy, sodium-restricted high protein diet, frequent urine protein monitoring |

[§] Complication or comorbid condition

# Albumin—
# Blood—Increased Level

Reference Range: 3.5-5.0

**Hospital Range:** _____

| Condition | Signs & Symptoms | Treatment |
|---|---|---|
| Dehydration[§] | Confusion, weakness, poor skin turgor, dry mucous membranes | Monitoring of electrolyte levels, intravenous therapy, force fluids, intake and output monitoring |

[§] Complication or comorbid condition

# Aldosterone— Blood—Increased Level

**Reference Range: 1-9**

**Hospital Range:** _____

| Condition | Signs & Symptoms | Treatment |
|---|---|---|
| **Failure, heart, congestive**[§†‡] | Peripheral edema, shortness of breath. Cyanosis is present on occasion. Heart rate is irregular, moist rales at base of lungs with productive cough. Confusion is usually present. | Sodium-restricted diet, digitalis regulation, $O_2$ therapy, diuretics |
| **Hypokalemia** | Nausea and vomiting, anorexia | Potassium supplement, intravenous fluids |

[§] Complication or comorbid condition
[†] Cardiovascular complication
[‡] Complex diagnosis

# Alkaline Phosphatase—
# Blood—Increased Level

**Reference Range: 25-70**

**Hospital Range:** _____

| Condition | Signs & Symptoms | Treatment |
|---|---|---|
| **Calculus of bile duct**[§] | Epigastric pain, nausea and vomiting, jaundice | Intravenous fluids and medications, surgery |
| **Cancer of liver**[§] | Weakness, fever, weight loss, right upper quadrant mass, pain | Chemotherapy, radiation, surgery |
| **Cirrhosis of liver**[§] | Abdominal pain or distention, fever, ascites, jaundice, anorexia | Sodium-restricted diet, intravenous fluids, treatment for relief of symptoms |
| **Leukemia**[§] | Weight loss, anorexia, pain in extremities, listlessness | Chemotherapy, intravenous fluids, transfusion(s) of blood and blood components, antibiotic therapy |
| **Pulmonary embolism**[§†‡] | Dyspnea, rales in lungs, sudden onset of substernal pain, dizziness, pallor | Heparin, diuretics |

[§] Complication or comorbid condition
[†] Cardiovascular complication
[‡] Complex diagnosis

# Amylase—
# Blood—Increased Level

**Reference Range: 60-160**

**Hospital Range:** _____

| Condition | Signs & Symptoms | Treatment |
|---|---|---|
| **Pancreatitis, acute**[§] | Epigastric pain, nausea, vomiting, fever, sweats, dizziness, confusion | Intravenous fluids, pain medication, replacement of calcium and magnesium if indicated |
| **Failure, renal, acute**[§] | Thirst, dyspnea, lethargy, weakness, anorexia, nausea | Management of diet, fluid and electrolytes. Possible dialysis |
| **Failure, renal, chronic**[§] | Bruising, dyspnea, lethargy, weakness, anorexia, polyuria | Fluid restrictions, dialysis, transfusion(s) of blood and blood components |
| **Ketoacidosis**[§] | Excessive thirst, polyuria, irritability, weakness | Restricted diet, monitoring of blood sugar levels |

[§] Complication or comorbid condition

# Arterial Blood Gases (ABGs)—
# Bicarbonate (HCO$_3$)—Decreased Level

**Reference Range: 24-28**

**Hospital Range:** _____

| Condition | Signs & Symptoms | Treatment |
|---|---|---|
| **Acidosis, metabolic**[§] | Hypotension, weakness, pallor, pulmonary edema | Fluid balance, electrolyte monitoring |
| **Failure, renal, chronic**[§] | Bruising, dyspnea, lethargy, weakness, anorexia, polyuria, hematuria | Fluid restrictions, dialysis, transfusion(s) of blood and blood components |
| **Infarction, acute myocardial**[§†] | Severe chest pain, gallop rhythm and other cardiac arrhythmias, shortness of breath, diaphoresis | Continuous monitoring, O$_2$ therapy, pain medication, intravenous fluids, intravenous medications, possible resuscitation |
| **Ketoacidosis**[§] | Excessive thirst, polyuria, irritability, weakness | Restricted diet, monitoring of blood sugar levels |

[§] Complication or comorbid condition
[†] Cardiovascular complication

# ABGs—pCO$_2$—
# Decreased Level

**Reference Range: 35-45**

**Hospital Range:** _____

| Condition | Signs & Symptoms | Treatment |
|-----------|------------------|-----------|
| **Acidosis, metabolic**[§] | Hypotension, weakness, pallor, pulmonary edema | Fluid balance, electrolyte monitoring |
| **Alkalosis, respiratory**[§] | Hyperventilation, hypoxia due to conditions such as sepsis, hyperventilation or drugs such as salicylates | Sedation, prevention of further hyperventilation |

[§] Complication or comorbid condition

*Abnormal Lab-9*

# ABGs—pCO$_2$—
# Increased Level

**Reference Range: 35-45**

**Hospital Range:** _____

| Condition | Signs & Symptoms | Treatment |
|---|---|---|
| **Alkalosis, metabolic**[§] | Nausea, vomiting, anorexia | Administration of aluminum chloride, respiratory therapy |
| **Alkalosis, respiratory**[§] | Retention of $CO_2$ and increasing $pCO_2$; hypoventilation, dyspnea, drowsiness, weakness, malaise and nausea due to conditions such as spinal cord injury, pulmonary disease or drugs such as narcotics | Establishment of airway, $O_2$ therapy, artificial ventilation, bicarbonate administration |
| **Disease, chronic obstructive pulmonary**[§] | Wheezing, productive cough, shortness of breath | Intermittent positive pressure breathing (IPPB) therapy, intravenous fluids, bronchodilators, antibiotics, physical therapy, artificial ventilation |

[§] Complication or comorbid condition

# ABGs—pH—
# Decreased Level

**Reference Range: 7.35-7.45**

**Hospital Range:** _____

| Condition | Signs & Symptoms | Treatment |
|---|---|---|
| **Acidosis, metabolic**[§] | Hypotension, weakness, pallor, pulmonary edema | Fluid balance, electrolyte monitoring |
| **Acidosis, respiratory**[§] | Retention of $CO_2$ and increasing $pCO_2$; hypoventilation, dyspnea, drowsiness, weakness, malaise and nausea due to conditions such as spinal cord injury, pulmonary disease or drugs such as narcotics | Establishment of airway, $O_2$ therapy, artificial ventilation, bicarbonate administration |
| **Ketoacidosis**[§] | Excessive thirst, polyuria, irritability, weakness, coma, stupor, dehydration, fruity breath odor | Restricted diet, monitoring of blood sugar levels, fluid replacement, insulin administration |

[§] Complication or comorbid condition

# ABGs—pO$_2$—
# Decreased Level

**Reference Range: 75-100**

**Hospital Range:** _____

| Condition | Signs & Symptoms | Treatment |
|---|---|---|
| **Disease, chronic obstructive pulmonary**[§] | Wheezing, productive cough, shortness of breath | IPPB therapy, intravenous fluids, bronchodilators, antibiotics, physical therapy, artificial ventilation |
| **Cor pulmonale, acute**[§‡] | Wheezing, marked fatigue, persistent cough, dyspnea | IPPB therapy, bronchodilators |
| **Edema, pulmonary**[§] | Increased respiration and pulse rate, shortness of breath, cough, anxiety, cyanosis, diaphoresis | Decreased rate of intravenous fluids, diuretics, intake and output monitoring, O$_2$ therapy, mechanical ventilation |

[§] Complication or comorbid condition
[†] Complex diagnosis

# Bilirubin—
# Indirect—Increased Level

**Reference Range: 0.1-1.0**

**Hospital Range:** _____

| Condition | Signs & Symptoms | Treatment |
|---|---|---|
| **Anemia, hemolytic** | Vomiting, anorexia, weight loss | Transfusion(s) of blood and blood components, chemotherapy, iron therapy, $O_2$ therapy |
| **Cirrhosis of liver**[§] | Abdominal pain or distention, fever, ascites, jaundice, anorexia | Sodium-restricted diet, intravenous fluids, treatment for relief of symptoms |
| **Failure, heart, congestive**[§††] | Peripheral edema, shortness of breath. Cyanosis is present on occasion. Heart rate is irregular, moist rales at base of lungs with productive cough. Confusion is usually present. | Sodium-restricted diet, digitalis regulation, $O_2$ therapy, diuretics |
| **Hyperbiliru-binemia (neonatal jaundice)** | Jaundice may be the only symptom as in physiologic jaundice. If caused by pathological jaundice, lack of treatment may result in kernicterus, a condition with severe neurological symptoms. | Phototherapy, exchange transfusion, administration of albumin |

[§] Complication or comorbid condition
[†] Cardiovascular complication
[‡] Complex diagnosis

# Bilirubin—
## Total/Direct—Increased Level

**Reference Range: 0.1-0.5 (D)**
                     **0.1-1.2 (T)**

**Hospital Range:** _____

| Condition | Signs & Symptoms | Treatment |
|---|---|---|
| **Calculus of bile duct**[§] | Epigastric pain, nausea and vomiting, jaundice | Intravenous fluids and medications, surgery |
| **Cancer of liver**[§] | Weakness, fever, weight loss, right upper quadrant mass, pain | Chemotherapy, radiation, surgery |
| **Cirrhosis of liver**[§] | Abdominal pain or distention, fever, ascites, jaundice, anorexia | Sodium-restricted diet, intravenous fluids, treatment for relief of symptoms |
| **Hepatitis**[§] | Jaundice, anorexia, dark urine, pruritus, light-colored stools | Rest, force fluids, antiemetics for nausea, isolation precautions for blood and other body fluids |

[§] Complication or comorbid condition

# Bleeding Time—
# Increased Level

**Reference Range: 2-10 minutes**

**Hospital Range:** _____

| Condition | Signs & Symptoms | Treatment |
|---|---|---|
| **Anemia, aplastic**[§] | Weakness, fatigue, shortness of breath | Reverse isolation, transfusion(s) of blood and blood components |
| **Coagulation, intravascular disseminated (DIC)**[§] | Occurs as a complication of other conditions such as infection, neoplastic disease, burns, and obstetric complications. Characterized by abnormal bleeding such as from the gastrointestinal tract and small wounds such as intravenous sites. Bruising is also present. | Transfusion of plasma or platelets; intravenous heparin administration; intake and output monitoring |
| **Disease, Von Willebrand's**[§] | Bruising, menorrhagia, epistaxis and possible hemorrhage as a result of surgery | Increased level of Factor VIII through infusion of cryoprecipitate or fresh frozen plasma prior to surgery or during bleeding episodes |

[§] Complication or comorbid condition

# Blood Urea Nitrogen (BUN)— Blood—Increased Level

**Reference Range: 9-22**

**Hospital Range:** _____

| Condition | Signs & Symptoms | Treatment |
|---|---|---|
| **Dehydration**[§] | Confusion, weakness, poor skin turgor, dry mucous membranes | Monitoring of electrolyte levels, intravenous therapy, force fluids, intake and output monitoring |
| **Infarction myocardial, acute**[§] | Severe chest pain, gallop rhythm and other cardiac arrhythmias, shortness of breath, diaphoresis | Continuous monitoring, $O_2$ therapy, pain medication, intravenous fluids, intravenous medications, possible resuscitation |
| **Failure, renal, acute**[§] | Thirst, dyspnea, lethargy, weakness, anorexia, nausea | Transfusion(s) of blood and blood components, dialysis, fluid restrictions |
| **Shock, cardiogenic**[§†‡] | Rapidly developing mental confusion, physical weakness, cold extremities, moist and cool skin, rapid and weak pulse, oliguria, pulmonary edema, hypotension | Fluid balance, $O_2$ therapy, cardiac monitoring |

[§] Complication or comorbid condition
[†] Cardiovascular complication
[‡] Complex diagnosis

# Calcium—
# Blood—Increased Level

**Reference Range: 8.5-10.5**

**Hospital Range:** _____

| Condition | Signs & Symptoms | Treatment |
|---|---|---|
| **Cancers that metastasize to bone**[§] | Lung and breast cancer | Surgery, chemotherapy, radiation therapy |
| **Failure, renal, acute**[§] | Thirst, dyspnea, lethargy, weakness, anorexia, nausea | Transfusion(s) of blood and blood components, dialysis, fluid restriction |
| **Hyperparathyroidism** | Muscle weakness, epigastric pain, recurrent renal calculi, hypertension | Hydration with intravenous saline, diuresis with furosemide, (lasix) surgery for parathyroid adenoma or hyperplasia |

[§] Complication or comorbid condition

# Carbon Dioxide ($CO_2$)—
# Decreased Level

**Reference Range: 22-30**

**Hospital Range:** _____

| Condition | Signs & Symptoms | Treatment |
|---|---|---|
| **Acidosis, metabolic**[§] | Hypotension, weakness, pallor, pulmonary edema | Fluid balance, electrolyte monitoring |
| **Dehydration**[§] | Confusion, weakness, poor skin turgor, dry mucous membranes | Monitoring of electrolyte levels, intravenous therapy, force fluids, intake and output monitoring |
| **Ketoacidosis**[§] | Excessive thirst, polyuria, weakness, irritability | Restricted diet, monitoring of blood sugar levels |

[§] Complication or comorbid condition

# Complete Blood Count (CBC)—
# Hematocrit (Hct)—Decreased Level

**Reference Range: Male 40-54%**
**Female 36-46%**

**Hospital Range:** _____

| Condition | Signs & Symptoms | Treatment |
|---|---|---|
| **Anemia, aplastic**[§] | Weakness, fatigue, shortness of breath | Reverse isolation, transfusion(s) of blood and blood components |
| **Anemia, hypochromic** | Tingling of extremities, dyspnea | Iron therapy, transfusion(s) of blood and blood components, $O_2$ therapy |
| **Cirrhosis of liver**[§] | Abdominal pain or distention, fever, ascites, jaundice, anorexia | Sodium-restricted diet, intravenous fluids, treatment for relief of symptoms |
| **Failure, chronic renal**[§] | Bruising, dyspnea, lethargy, weakness, anorexia, polyuria, hematuria | Sodium-restricted diet, digitalis regulation, $O_2$ therapy, diuretics |
| **Hemorrhage, not otherwise specified**[§] | Pallor, rapid and shallow respirations, unstable vital signs, melena, hemoptysis, weakness | Intravenous therapy, transfusion(s) of blood and blood components, vitamin K, iron therapy |
| **Leukemia**[§] | Weight loss, anorexia, pain in extremities, listlessness | Chemotherapy, intravenous fluids, transfusion(s) of blood and blood components, antibiotic therapy |

[§] Complication or comorbid condition

# CBC—
# Hematocrit (Hct)—Increased Level

**Reference Range: Male 40-54%**
**Female 36-46%**

**Hospital Range:** _____

| Condition | Signs & Symptoms | Treatment |
|---|---|---|
| Dehydration[§] | Confusion, weakness, poor skin turgor, dry mucous membranes | Monitoring of electrolyte levels, intravenous therapy, force fluids, intake and output monitoring |
| Disease, chronic obstructive pulmonary[§] | Wheezing, productive cough, shortness of breath | IPPB therapy, intravenous fluids, bronchodilators, antibiotics, physical therapy, artificial ventilation |
| Polycythemia vera | Fatigue, pruritis, vertigo, dizziness, cerebrovascular accident (CVA), transient ischemic attack (TIA) | Phlebotomy |
| Shock, hypovolemic[§] | Cold clammy skin, tachycardia, shallow respirations, hypotension, weak thready pulse, confusion | Intravenous therapy, frequent monitoring of vital signs, intake and output monitoring |

[§] Complication or comorbid condition

# CBC—
# Hemoglobin (Hgb)—Decreased Level

**Reference Range: Male 13.5-18**
**Female 12-16**

**Hospital Range:** _____

| Condition | Signs & Symptoms | Treatment |
|---|---|---|
| **Anemia, aplastic**[§] | Weakness, fatigue, shortness of breath | Reverse isolation, transfusion(s) of blood and blood components |
| **Anemia, hypochromic** | Tingling of extremities, dyspnea | Iron therapy, transfusion(s) of blood and blood components, $O_2$ therapy |
| **Cancer: Large Intestine**[§] | Pain, change in bowel or bladder habit, diarrhea, constipation | Chemotherapy, radiation therapy, surgery |
| **Liver**[§] | Melena, weight loss, clay-colored stools, digestive disturbances | Chemotherapy, radiation therapy, surgery |
| **Rectum**[§] | Pain, incomplete bowel movement, bleeding of rectum | Chemotherapy, radiation therapy, surgery |
| **Small intestine**[§] | Weight loss, vomiting, fever, chills, melena | Chemotherapy, radiation therapy, surgery |
| **Cirrhosis of liver**[§] | Abdominal pain or distention, fever, ascites, jaundice, anorexia, polyuria | Sodium-restricted diet, intravenous fluids, treatment for relief of symptoms |
| **Failure, chronic renal**[§] | Bruising, dyspnea, lethargy, weakness, anorexia, polyuria, hematuria | Fluid restrictions, dialysis, transfusion(s) of blood and blood components |

*continued*

[§] Complication or comorbid condition

*Abnormal Lab-21*

# CBC—
# Hemoglobin (Hgb)—Decreased Level
## *continued*

**Reference Range: Male 13.5-18**
**Female 12-16**

**Hospital Range:** _____

| Condition | Signs & Symptoms | Treatment |
|---|---|---|
| **Hemorrhage, not otherwise specified**[§] | Pallor, rapid and shallow respirations, unstable vital signs, melena, hemoptysis, weakness, hematemesis | Intravenous therapy, vitamin K, iron therapy, transfusion(s) of blood and blood components |
| **Kidney disease** | Lethargy, weakness, nausea and vomiting, thirst, dyspnea, convulsions | Transfusion(s) of blood and blood components, dialysis, fluid restrictions |
| **Leukemia**[§] | Weight loss, anorexia, pain in extremities, listlessness | Chemotherapy, intravenous fluids, transfusion(s) of blood and blood components, antibiotic therapy |

[§] Complication or comorbid condition

# CBC—
# Hemoglobin (Hgb)—Increased Level

**Reference Range: Male 13.5-18**
**Female 12-16**

**Hospital Range:** _____

| Condition | Signs & Symptoms | Treatment |
|---|---|---|
| **Dehydration**[§] | Confusion, weakness, poor skin turgor, dry mucous membranes | Monitoring of electrolyte levels, intravenous therapy, force fluids, intake and output monitoring |
| **Disease, chronic obstructive pulmonary**[§] | Wheezing, productive cough, shortness of breath | IPPB therapy, intravenous fluids, bronchodilators, antibiotics, physical therapy, artificial ventilation |
| **Failure, congestive heart**[§‡] | Peripheral edema, shortness of breath. Cyanosis is present on occasion. Heart rate is irregular, moist rales at base of lungs with productive cough. Confusion usually present. Paroxysmal nocturnal dyspnea, wheezing. | Sodium-restricted diet, digitalis regulation, $O_2$ therapy, diuretics |

[§] Complication or comorbid condition
[‡] Complex diagnosis

# CBC—
# Mean Corpuscular Hemoglobin (MCH)
# Decreased Level

**Reference Range: 27-31**

**Hospital Range:** _____

| Condition | Signs & Symptoms | Treatment |
|---|---|---|
| **Anemia, hypo-chromic** | Tingling of extremities, dyspnea | Iron therapy, transfusion(s) of blood and blood components, $O_2$ therapy |
| **Hemorrhage, not otherwise specified**[§] | Pallor, rapid and shallow respirations, unstable vital signs, melena, hemoptysis, weakness | Intravenous therapy, transfusion(s) of blood and blood components, vitamin K, iron therapy |

[§] Complication or comorbid condition

# CBC—
# Mean Corpuscular
# Hemoglobin Concentration (MCHC)—
# Decreased Level

**Reference Range: 32-36%**

**Hospital Range:** _____

| Condition | Signs & Symptoms | Treatment |
|-----------|------------------|-----------|
| **Anemia, hypo-chromic** | Tingling of extremities, dyspnea | Iron therapy, transfusion(s) of blood and blood compo-nents, $O_2$ therapy |
| **Thalassemia**[§] | Depending on type, symptoms range from severe anemia, skeletal malformation, hepatome-galy and bleeding tenden-cies to mild anemia. | Folic acid supplements, transfusion of packed red blood cells |

[§] Complication or comorbid condition

# CBC—
# Mean Corpuscular Volume (MCV)—
# Decreased Level

**Reference Range: Male 80-94**
**Female 78-97**

**Hospital Range:** _____

| Condition | Signs & Symptoms | Treatment |
|---|---|---|
| **Anemia, hypo-chromic** | Tingling of extremities, dyspnea | Iron therapy, transfusion(s) of blood and blood components, $O_2$ therapy |
| **Failure, chronic renal**[§] | Bruising, dyspnea, lethargy, weakness, anorexia, polyuria, hematuria | Fluid restrictions, dialysis, transfusion(s) of blood and blood components |
| **Thalassemia**[§] | Depending on type, symptoms range from severe anemia, skeletal malformation, hepatomegaly and bleeding tendencies to mild anemia. | Folic acid supplements, transfusion of packed red blood cells |

[§] Complication or comorbid condition

# CBC—Red Blood Count (RBC)— Decreased Level

**Reference Range: Male 4.4-6.0**
**Female 4.2-5.5**

**Hospital Range:** _____

| Condition | Signs & Symptoms | Treatment |
|---|---|---|
| **Aplastic anemia**[§] | Weakness, fatigue, shortness of breath | Reverse isolation, transfusion(s) of blood and blood components |
| **Anemia, posthemorrhagic**[§] | Weight loss, weakness, pain, anorexia | $B_{12}$, folic acid supplement, iron therapy, transfusion(s) of blood and blood components |
| **Failure, chronic renal**[§] | Bruising, dyspnea, lethargy, weakness, anorexia, polyuria, hematuria | Fluid restrictions, dialysis, transfusion(s) of blood and blood components |
| **Hemorrhage, not otherwise specified**[§] | Pallor, rapid and shallow breathing, unstable vital signs, melena, hemoptysis, weakness | Intravenous therapy, transfusion(s) of blood and blood components, vitamin K, iron therapy |
| **Overhydration**[§] | Irritability, weakness, muscle cramps | Restriction of fluid intake |

[§] Complication or comorbid condition

# CBC—RBC—
# Increased Level

**Reference Range: Male 4.4-6.0**
**Female 4.2-5.5**

**Hospital Range:** _____

| Condition | Signs & Symptoms | Treatment |
|---|---|---|
| **Cor pulmonale, acute**[§‡] | Wheezing, marked fatigue, persistent cough, dyspnea | IPPB therapy, bronchodilators |
| **Dehydration**[§] | Confusion, weakness, poor skin turgor, dry mucous membranes | Monitoring of electrolyte levels, intravenous therapy, force fluids, intake and output monitoring |
| **Polycythemia vera** | Fatigue, pruritis, vertigo, dizziness, CVA, TIA | Phlebotomy |

[§] Complication or comorbid condition
[‡] Complex diagnosis

# CBC—
# White Blood Count (WBC)—
# Above 10,000

**Reference Range: 5,000-10,000**

**Hospital Range:** _____

| Condition | Signs & Symptoms | Treatment |
|---|---|---|
| **Chronic renal failure**[§] | Bruising, dyspnea, lethargy, weakness, anorexia, polyuria | Fluid restrictions, dialysis, transfusion(s) of blood and blood components |
| **Cirrhosis of liver**[§] | Abdominal pain or distention, fever, ascites, jaundice, anorexia | Sodium-restricted diet, intravenous fluids, treatment for relief of symptoms |
| **Embolism, pulmonary**[§†‡] | Dyspnea, rales in lungs, sudden onset of substernal pain, dizziness, pallor, hemoptysis | Heparin, diuretics |
| **Failure, renal acute**[§†] | Thirst, dyspnea, lethargy, weakness, anorexia, nausea and vomiting | Management of diet, fluid, electrolytes. Possible dialysis |
| **Infarction, myocardial acute**[§†] | Severe chest pain, gallop rhythm and other cardiac arrhythmias, shortness of breath, diaphoresis | Continuous monitoring, $O_2$ therapy, pain medication, intravenous fluids, intravenous medications, possible resuscitation, drug therapy |
| **Infections, acute** | Fever, malaise, chills | Intravenous fluids, antibiotic therapy |
| **Leukemia**[§] | Weight loss, anorexia, pain in extremities, listlessness | Chemotherapy, intravenous fluids, transfusion(s) of blood and blood components, antibiotic therapy |

*continued*

[§] Complication or comorbid condition
[†] Cardiovascular complication
[‡] Complex diagnosis

# CBC—
# White Blood Count (WBC)—Above 10,000
## *continued*

**Reference Range: 5,000-10,000**

**Hospital Range:** _____

| Condition | Signs & Symptoms | Treatment |
|---|---|---|
| Leukocytosis | Increase in the number of leukocytes in the blood. Can result from hemorrhage, inflammation or infection. | Diagnostic investigations to determine cause of leukocytosis |
| Pneumonia[§] | Dyspnea, chills, chest pain, cough, fever, headache | Intravenous fluids, $O_2$ therapy, antibiotic therapy |
| Pneumonia, aspiration[§] | Cyanosis, cough, dyspnea | Intravenous fluids, $O_2$ therapy, antibiotic therapy |
| Pneumonia, pneumococcal[§] | Cough, severe chest pain, shortness of breath | Intravenous fluids, $O_2$ therapy, antibiotic therapy |
| Pneumonia, E.coli/proteus[§] | Chest pain, shortness of breath, malaise | Intravenous fluids, $O_2$ therapy, antibiotic therapy |
| Pneumonia, staphylococcal[§] | Headache, chest pain, cough | Intravenous fluids, $O_2$ therapy, antibiotic therapy |
| Pyelonephritis[§] | Nausea and vomiting, frequency of urination, dysuria, flank pain, chills | Sulfonimides, intravenous fluids, force fluids, antibiotic therapy |
| Urinary tract infection[§] | Fever, dysuria, frequency, burning on urination, hematuria | Urinary antiseptics, antibiotic therapy, intravenous fluids, force fluids |

[§] Complication or comorbid condition
[†] Cardiovascular complication
[‡] Complex diagnosis

# CBC—
# WBC—Below 5,000

**Reference Range: 5,000-10,000**

**Hospital Range:** _____

| Condition | Signs & Symptoms | Treatment |
|---|---|---|
| **Anemia, aplastic**[§] | Weakness, fatigue, shortness of breath, bruising, nosebleeds | Reverse isolation, transfusion(s) of blood and blood components |
| **Leukopenia**[§] | Headache, weakness, shortness of breath on exertion | Transfusion(s) of blood and blood components, intravenous fluids |

[§] Complication or comorbid condition

# Chloride (Cl)—
# Blood, Electrolytes—Decreased Level

**Reference Range: 95-105**

**Hospital Range:** _____

| Condition | Signs & Symptoms | Treatment |
|---|---|---|
| **Burns** | Can result from thermal, electrical or chemical injuries. Severity is estimated by the size and depth of the burn | Reverse isolation, skin grafts, intravenous fluids, invasive monitoring, high protein/high calorie diet |
| **Hypo-natremia**[§] | Weakness, muscle cramps and spasms, confusion, irritability | Intravenous fluids, sodium concentrate |
| **Ketoacidosis**[§] | Irritability, weakness, excessive thirst, polyuria | Restricted diet, monitoring of blood sugar levels |

[§] Complication or comorbid condition

# Chloride (Cl)—
# Blood, Electrolytes—Increased Level

**Reference Range: 95-105**

**Hospital Range:** _____

| Condition | Signs & Symptoms | Treatment |
|---|---|---|
| **Acidosis, metabolic**[§] | Hypotension, weakness, pallor, pulmonary edema | Fluid balance, electrolyte monitoring |
| **Dehydration**[§] | Confusion, weakness, poor skin turgor, dry mucous membranes | Monitoring of electrolyte levels, intravenous therapy, force fluids, intake and output monitoring |
| **Failure, renal, acute**[§] | Thirst, dyspnea, lethargy, weakness, anorexia, nausea | Management of diet, fluid and electrolytes; possible dialysis |
| **Hyper-natremia**[§] | Poor skin turgor, dry mucous membranes, confusion, stupor, coma | Intravenous fluids, force fluids, administration of $H_2O$ |

[§] Complication or comorbid condition

# Cholesterol—
# Increased Level

**Reference Range: 150-250**

**Hospital Range:** _____

| Condition | Signs & Symptoms | Treatment |
|---|---|---|
| **Calculus of bile duct**[§] | Epigastric pain and nausea, vomiting, jaundice | Intravenous fluids and medications, surgery |
| **Cirrhosis of liver**[§] | Abdominal pain or distention, fever, ascites, jaundice, anorexia | Sodium-restricted diet, intravenous fluids, treatment for relief of symptoms |
| **Diabetes mellitus, out of control**[§] | Excessive thirst, polyuria, irritability, weakness | Restricted diet, monitoring of blood sugar levels, treatment for symptomatology |
| **Failure, renal, acute**[§] | Thirst, dyspnea, lethargy, weakness, anorexia, nausea | Transfusion(s) of blood and blood components, dialysis, fluid restriction |
| **Infarction, myocardial acute**[§] | Severe chest pain, gallop rhythm and other cardiac arrhythmias, shortness of breath, diaphoresis | Continuous monitoring, $O_2$ therapy, pain medication, intravenous fluids, intravenous medications, possible resuscitation |

[§] Complication or comorbid condition

# Cold Agglutinins—
# Increased Level

**Reference Range: 1:15 Tite or less**

**Hospital Range:** _____

| Condition | Signs & Symptoms | Treatment |
|---|---|---|
| **Anemia, hemolytic** | Vomiting, anorexia, weight loss | Transfusion(s) of blood and blood components, chemotherapy, iron and $O_2$ therapy |
| **Cirrhosis of liver**[§] | Abdominal pain or distention, fever, ascites, anorexia | Sodium-restricted diet, intravenous fluids, treatment for relief of symptoms |
| **Hepatitis**[§] | Jaundice, anorexia, dark urine, pruritus, light-colored stools | Rest, force fluids, anti-emetics for nausea, isolation precautions for blood and other body fluids |
| **Pneumonia**[§] | Dyspnea, chills, chest pain, cough, fever, headache | Intravenous fluids, $O_2$ therapy, antibiotic therapy |

[§] Complication or comorbid condition

# Creatinine—
# Blood—Increased Level

**Reference Range: 0.6-1.2**

**Hospital Range:** _____

| Condition | Signs & Symptoms | Treatment |
|-----------|------------------|-----------|
| **Failure, renal, acute**[§] | Thirst, dyspnea, lethargy, weakness, anorexia, nausea | Management of diet, fluid and electrolytes; possible dialysis |
| **Glomerulo-nephritis, chronic** | Hypertension, hematuria, azotemia, fatigue | Diuretics, dietary restrictions, antibiotics, dialysis or surgical transplantation |
| **Infection, urinary tract**[§] | Fever, dysuria, frequency, burning on urination | Urinary antiseptics, antibiotic therapy, intravenous fluids, force fluids |

[§] Complication or comorbid condition

# Creatinine Phosphokinase (CPK) (CK)— Blood—Increased Level

**Reference Range: 21-232**

**Hospital Range:** _____

| Condition | Signs & Symptoms | Treatment |
|---|---|---|
| **Infarction, myocardial, acute**[§] | Severe chest pain, gallop rhythm and other cardiac arrhythmias, shortness of breath, diaphoresis | Continuous monitoring, $O_2$ therapy, pain medication, intravenous fluids, intravenous medications, possible resuscitation |
| **Muscular dystrophy**[§] | Predominant symptom is weakness. As disease progresses, muscle atrophy, abnormal gait and cardiac symptoms, such as tachycardia, appear. | Physical therapy, orthopaedic appliances, surgery to release contractures |
| **Pulmonary embolism**[§†‡] | Dyspnea, rales in lungs, sudden onset of substernal pain, dizziness, pallor | Heparin, diuretics |

[§] Complication or comorbid condition
[†] Cardiovascular complication
[‡] Complex diagnosis

# Creatinine Phosphokinase MB-Fraction (CPK-MB) (CK-MB)— Increased Level

**Reference Range: 21-232**

**Hospital Range:** _____

| Condition | Signs & Symptoms | Treatment |
|---|---|---|
| Infarction, myocardial, acute[§] | Severe chest pain, gallop rhythm and other cardiac arrhythmias, shortness of breath, diaphoresis | Continuous monitoring, $O_2$ therapy, pain medication, intravenous fluids, intravenous medications, possible resuscitation |
| Muscular dystrophy[§] | Predominant symptom is weakness. As disease progresses, muscle atrophy, abnormal gait and cardiac symptoms, such as tachycardia, appear. | Physical therapy, orthopaedic appliances, surgery to release contractures |

[§] Complication or comorbid condition

# White Blood Cell Differential (WBC-DIFF)— Basophils—Increased Level

**Reference Range: 0.4-1%**

**Hospital Range:** _____

| Condition | Signs & Symptoms | Treatment |
|---|---|---|
| **Anemia, hemolytic** | Vomiting, anorexia, weight loss | Transfusion(s) of blood and blood components, chemotherapy, iron therapy, $O_2$ therapy |
| **Leukemia**[§] | Weight loss, anorexia, pain in extremities, listlessness | Chemotherapy, intravenous fluids, transfusion(s) of blood and blood components, antibiotic therapy |
| **Polycythemia vera** | Fatigue, pruritis, vertigo, dizziness, CVA, TIA | Phlebotomy, radiophosphorus (32P) |

[§] Complication or comorbid condition

# Differential (WBC-DIFF)— Eosinophils—Increased Level

**Reference Range: 1-3%**

**Hospital Range:** _____

| Condition | Signs & Symptoms | Treatment |
|-----------|------------------|-----------|
| **Cancer, lung** | Cough, dyspnea, chest and shoulder pain, fever, weight loss, hemoptysis | Surgery, chemotherapy, radiation therapy |
| **Disease, Addison's**[§] | Features of crisis include anorexia, headache, weakness, nausea, vomiting, apprehension, diarrhea, abdominal pain, syncope. Chronic Addison's disease may show indications resembling hypoglycemia (i.e., hunger, sweating, irritability, nervousness, depression). | Glucocorticoid and mineralocorticoid replacement |
| **Leukemia**[§] | Weight loss, anorexia, pain in extremities, listlessness | Chemotherapy, intravenous fluids, transfusion(s) of blood and blood components, antibiotic therapy |
| **Parasitism, intestinal** | Diarrhea, abdominal pain, nausea and vomiting | Fluid replacement (intravenous or by mouth), antibiotics, symptomatic treatment, such as Kaopectate |
| **Reaction, allergic** | Can assume a variety of forms from contact dermatitis to anaphylactic shock. Most reactions occur on the skin or in the respiratory or gastrointestinal tract. | Maintenance of airway, epinephrine, aminophylline |

[§] Complication or comorbid condition

# Differential (WBC-DIFF)—
## Lymphocytes—Decreased Level

**Reference Range: 25-35%**

**Hospital Range:** _____

| Condition | Signs & Symptoms | Treatment |
|---|---|---|
| **Anemia, aplastic**[§] | Weakness, fatigue, shortness of breath | Reverse isolation, transfusion(s) of blood and blood components |
| **Burns** | Can result from thermal, electrical or chemical injuries. Severity is estimated by depth and size of burn. | Reverse isolation, skin grafts, intravenous fluids, invasive monitoring, high protein/high calorie diet |
| **Disease, Hodgkin's** [§] | Lymphadenopathy, infections, purpura, fatigue | Reverse isolation, radiation therapy, chemotherapy |
| **Lymphocytopenia** | Can result from radiation or chemotherapy, renal failure or terminal cancer. Symptoms include enlarged lymph nodes and spleen. | Treatment of underlying condition; reverse isolation |

[§] Complication or comorbid condition

# Differential (WBC-DIFF)— Lymphocytes—Increased Level

**Reference Range: 25-35%**

**Hospital Range:** _____

| Condition | Signs & Symptoms | Treatment |
|---|---|---|
| **Leukemia**[§] | Weight loss, anorexia, pain in extremities, listlessness | Chemotherapy, intravenous fluids, transfusion(s) of blood and blood components, antibiotic therapy |
| **Leukemia, acute lymphoblastic**[§] | Lymphadenopathy, infections, purpura, fatigue | Reverse isolation, chemotherapy, bone marrow transplantation |
| **Lymphocytosis** | May be relative or absolute. Associated with bacterial and viral conditions such as mumps, measles and tuberculosis. Infectious lymphocytosis is a mild childhood disease. | Treatment of underlying condition |
| **Mononucleosis, infectious** | Fever, lymphadenopathy, fatigue | Bed rest, antibiotics, aspirin or acetaminophen for discomfort |
| **Pneumonia**[§] | Dyspnea, chills, chest pain, cough, fever, headache | Intravenous fluids, $O_2$ therapy, antibiotic therapy |

[§] Complication or comorbid condition

# Differential (WBC-DIFF)— Segmented Neutrophils (Segs)— Decreased Level

**Reference Range: 51-67%**

**Hospital Range:** _____

| Condition | Signs & Symptoms | Treatment |
|---|---|---|
| **Anemia, aplastic**[§] | Weakness, fatigue, shortness of breath | Reverse isolation, transfusion(s) of blood and blood components |
| **Disease, Addison's** | Features of crisis include anorexia, headache, weakness, nausea, vomiting, apprehension, diarrhea, abdominal pain, syncope. Chronic Addison's disease may show indications resembling hypoglycemia (i.e., hunger, sweating, irritability, nervousness, depression). | Glucocorticoid and mineralocorticoid replacement |

[§] Complication or comorbid condition

# Differential (WBC-DIFF)—
# Segmented Neutrophils (Segs)—
# Increased Level

**Reference Range: 51-67%**

**Hospital Range:** _____

| Condition | Signs & Symptoms | Treatment |
|---|---|---|
| **Infarction, acute myocardial**[§] | Severe chest pain, gallop rhythm and other cardiac arrhythmias, shortness of breath, diaphoresis | Continuous monitoring, $O_2$ therapy, pain medication, intravenous fluids, intravenous medications, possible resuscitation |
| **Leukemia**[§] | Weight loss, anorexia, pain in extremities, listlessness | Chemotherapy, intravenous fluids, transfusion(s) of blood and blood components, antibiotic therapy |
| **Pneumonia**[§] | Dyspnea, chills, chest pain, cough, fever, headache | Intravenous fluids, $O_2$ therapy, antibiotic therapy |

[§] Complication or comorbid condition

# Gamma Glutamyl Transferase (GT, GGT)—
# Increased Level

**Reference Range: 10-38**

**Hospital Range:** _____

| Condition | Signs & Symptoms | Treatment |
|---|---|---|
| **Alcoholism**[§] | Inability to control alcohol consumption. Symptoms can include maladaptive behavior, flushed face and delirium tremens (DTs). | Antianxiety drugs, B vitamins, psychotherapy |
| **Calculus of bile duct**[§] | Epigastric pain, nausea and vomiting, jaundice | Intravenous fluids and medications, surgery |
| **Cirrhosis of liver**[§] | Abdominal pain or distention, fever, ascites, jaundice, anorexia | Sodium-restricted diet, intravenous fluids, treatment for relief of symptoms |
| **Pancreatitis, acute**[§] | Epigastric pain, nausea, vomiting, fever, sweats, dizziness, confusion | Intravenous fluids, pain medication, replacement of calcium and magnesium if indicated |

[§]Complication or comorbid condition

# Glucose (Fasting Blood Sugar (FBS))—
# Blood—Decreased Level

**Reference Range: 70-115**

**Hospital Range:** _____

| Condition | Signs & Symptoms | Treatment |
|---|---|---|
| **Cancer of pancreas**§ | Diarrhea, weight loss, abdominal pain, jaundice, nausea, anorexia | Surgery, chemotherapy, radiation therapy |
| **Failure, renal, chronic**§ | Bruising, dyspnea, lethargy, weakness, anorexia, polyuria | Fluid restrictions, dialysis, transfusion(s) of blood and blood components |
| **Hepatitis**§ | Jaundice, anorexia, dark urine, pruritus, light-colored stools | Rest, force fluids, antiemetics for nausea, isolation precautions for blood and other body fluids |
| **Reaction, hypoglycemia**§ | Sudden onset of sweating, pale skin, blurred vision, possible loss of consciousness | Withheld insulin, food or juice given with sugar, glucose injection |

§ Complication or comorbid condition

# Glucose (FBS)—
# Blood—Increased Level

**Reference Range: 70-115**

**Hospital Range:** _____

| Condition | Signs & Symptoms | Treatment |
|---|---|---|
| **Diabetes mellitus, out of control**[§] | Excessive thirst, polyuria, irritability, weakness | Diet restriction, monitoring of blood sugar, treatment for symptomatology |
| **Failure, heart, congestive**[§†‡] | Peripheral edema, shortness of breath. Cyanosis is present on occasion. Heart rate is irregular, moist rales at base of lungs with productive cough. Confusion is usually present. | Sodium-restricted diet, digitalis regulation, $O_2$ therapy, diuretics |
| **Failure, renal, acute**[§] | Thirst, dyspnea, lethargy, weakness, anorexia, nausea | Transfusion(s) of blood and blood components, dialysis, fluid restrictions |
| **Infarction, myocardial, acute**[§] | Severe chest pain, gallop rhythm and other cardiac arrhythmias, shortness of breath, diaphoresis | Continuous monitoring, $O_2$ therapy, pain medication, intravenous fluids, intravenous medications, possible resuscitation |
| **Infections (acute)** | Fever, malaise, chills | Intravenous fluids, antibiotic therapy |
| **Ketoacidosis**[§] | Irritability, weakness, excessive thirst, polyuria | Restricted diet, monitoring of blood sugar levels |

[§] Complication or comorbid condition
[†] Cardiovascular complication
[‡] Complex diagnosis

# Lactic Dehydrogenase (LDH) (LD)— Increased Level

**Reference Range: 100-190**

**Hospital Range:** _____

| Condition | Signs & Symptoms | Treatment |
|---|---|---|
| **Cirrhosis of liver**[§] | Abdominal pain or distention, fever, ascites, jaundice, anorexia | Sodium-restricted diet, intravenous fluids, treatment for relief of symptoms |
| **Failure, heart, congestive**[§†‡] | Peripheral edema, shortness of breath. Cyanosis is present on occasion. Heart rate is irregular, moist rales at base of lungs with productive cough. Confusion is usually present. | Sodium-restricted diet, digitalis regulation, $O_2$ therapy, diuretics |
| **Hemolytic anemia** | Vomiting, anorexia, weight loss | Transfusion(s) of blood and blood components, chemotherapy, iron therapy, $O_2$ therapy |
| **Infarction, myocardial, acute**[§] | Severe chest pain, gallop rhythm and other cardiac arrhythmias, shortness of breath, diaphoresis | Continuous monitoring, $O_2$ therapy, pain medication, intravenous fluids, intravenous medications, possible resuscitation |
| **Pernicious anemia** | Paresthesia, weakness, nausea, vomiting, ataxia | Parenteral administration of $B_{12}$ |
| **Pulmonary embolism**[§†‡] | Dyspnea, rales in lungs, sudden onset of substernal pain, dizziness, pallor | Heparin, diuretics |

[§] Complication or comorbid condition
[†] Cardiovascular complication
[‡] Complex diagnosis

# Lactic Dehydrogenase-1 (LD-1)— Increased Level

**Reference Range: 40-65**

**Hospital Range:** _____

| Condition | Signs & Symptoms | Treatment |
|---|---|---|
| **Anemia, hemolytic** | Vomiting, anorexia, weight loss | Transfusion(s) of blood and blood components, chemotherapy, iron therapy, $O_2$ therapy |
| **Anemia, megaloblastic** | Paresthesia, ataxia, memory loss | Parenteral administration of $B_{12}$; folic acid supplements |
| **Infarction, myocardial, acute[§]** | Severe chest pain, gallop rhythm and other cardiac arrhythmias, shortness of breath, diaphoresis | Continuous monitoring, $O_2$ therapy, pain medication, intravenous fluids, intravenous medications, possible resuscitation |

[§] Complication or comorbid condition

# Lipase—
# Increased Level

**Reference Range: 0-1.5**

**Hospital Range:** _____

| Condition | Signs & Symptoms | Treatment |
|---|---|---|
| **Cirrhosis of liver**[§] | Abdominal pain or distention, fever, ascites, jaundice, anorexia | Sodium-restricted diet, intravenous fluids, treatment for relief of symptoms |
| **Failure, renal, acute**[§] | Thirst, dyspnea, lethargy, weakness, anorexia, nausea | Management of diet, fluid and electrolytes; possible dialysis |
| **Pancreatitis, acute**[§] | Epigastric pain, nausea, vomiting, fever, sweats, dizziness, confusion | Intravenous fluids, pain medication, replacement of calcium and magnesium if indicated |

[§] Complication or comorbid condition

# Magnesium—
# Blood—Increased Level

**Reference Range: 1.5-2.5**

**Hospital Range:** _____

| Condition | Signs & Symptoms | Treatment |
|---|---|---|
| **Dehydration**[§] | Confusion, weakness, poor skin turgor, dry mucous membranes | Monitoring of electrolyte levels, intravenous therapy, force fluids, intake and output monitoring |
| **Failure, renal, chronic**[§] | Bruising, dyspnea, lethargy, weakness, anorexia, polyuria | Fluid restrictions, dialysis, transfusion(s) of blood and blood components |
| **Leukemia**[§] | Weight loss, anorexia, pain in extremities, listlessness | Chemotherapy, intravenous fluids, transfusion(s) of blood and blood components, antibiotic therapy |

[§] Complication or comorbid condition

# Osmolality—
# Blood—Decreased Level

**Reference Range: 280-300**

**Hospital Range:** _____

| Condition | Signs & Symptoms | Treatment |
|---|---|---|
| **Cancer of bronchus**[§] | Productive cough, shortness of breath, dyspnea | Chemotherapy, intravenous fluids |
| **Cancer of lung**[§] | Congestion, shortness of breath, productive cough | Chemotherapy, intravenous fluids, surgery, radiation therapy |
| **Deficiency, ADH**[§] | Polydipsia, polyuria, headaches, fatigue | Antidiuretic hormone replacement therapy, intake and output monitoring, daily weights |
| **Hypona-tremia**[§] | Weakness, muscle cramps and spasms, confusion, anorexia, nausea | Intravenous fluids, sodium concentrate |

[§] Complication or comorbid condition

# Osmolality—
# Blood—Increased Level

**Reference Range: 280-300**

**Hospital Range:** _____

| Condition | Signs & Symptoms | Treatment |
|---|---|---|
| **Cirrhosis of liver**[§] | Abdominal pain or distention, fever, ascites, jaundice, anorexia | Sodium-restricted diet, intravenous fluids, treatment for relief of symptoms |
| **Dehydration**[§] | Confusion, weakness, poor skin turgor, dry mucous membranes | Monitoring of electrolyte levels, intravenous therapy, force fluids, intake and output monitoring |
| **Hyper-natremia**[§] | Irritability, lethargy, weakness, confusion, stupor, coma | Intravenous fluids, force fluids, administration of $H_2O$ |

[§] Complication or comorbid condition

# Platelet Count— Decreased Level

**Reference Range: 150,000-400,000**

**Hospital Range:** _____

| Condition | Signs & Symptoms | Treatment |
|---|---|---|
| **Anemia, aplastic**[§] | Weakness, fatigue, shortness of breath | Reverse isolation, transfusion(s) of blood and blood components |
| **Disease, kidney** | Lethargy, weakness, nausea and vomiting, thirst, dyspnea, convulsions | Transfusion(s) of blood and blood components, dialysis, fluid restrictions |
| **Leukemia**[§] | Weight loss, anorexia, pain in extremities, listlessness | Chemotherapy, intravenous fluids, transfusion(s) of blood and blood components, antibiotic therapy |
| **Reaction, drug, to antineoplastic agents and other medications such as heparin** | Spontaneous bleeding such as bruising, epistaxis and gastrointestinal bleeding | Discontinuation of offending drug; platelet transfusion for acute hemorrhage |
| **Thrombocytopenia**[§] | Can be due to decreased production of platelets or increased destruction. Symptoms include spontaneous bleeding in the skin or any mucous membrane. | Treatment of underlying condition. May include corticosteroids and transfusion of blood and blood components, such as platelets |

[§] Complication or comorbid condition

# Platelet Count—
# Increased Level

**Reference Range: 150,000-400,000**

**Hospital Range:** _____

| Condition | Signs & Symptoms | Treatment |
|---|---|---|
| **Cirrhosis of liver**[§] | Abdominal pain or distention, fever, ascites, jaundice, anorexia | Sodium-restricted diet, intravenous fluids, treatment for relief of symptoms |
| **Hemorrhage, not otherwise specified**[§] | Pallor, rapid and shallow respirations, unstable vital signs, melena, hemoptysis, weakness | Intravenous therapy, transfusion(s) of blood and blood components, vitamin K, iron therapy |
| **Infections (acute)** | Fever, malaise, chills | Intravenous fluids, antibiotic therapy |
| **Thrombocy-tosis** | Can occur as a result of many conditions such as trauma, cancer, anemia and heart disease. | Treatment of underlying condition |

[§] Complication or comorbid condition

# Potassium (K)—
# Blood—Decreased Level

**Reference Range: 3.5-5.0**

**Hospital Range:** _____

| Condition | Signs & Symptoms | Treatment |
|---|---|---|
| **Dehydration**[§] | Confusion, weakness, poor skin turgor, dry mucous membranes | Monitoring of electrolyte levels, intravenous therapy, force fluids, intake and output monitoring |
| **Failure, renal, acute**[§] | Thirst, dyspnea, lethargy, weakness, anorexia, nausea | Management of diet, fluid and electrolytes; possible dialysis |
| **Hypokalemia**[§] | Cardiac arrhythmias, leg cramps, nausea and vomiting | Administration of potassium chloride orally or intravenously |
| **Ketoacidosis**[§] | Irritability, weakness, excessive thirst, polyuria | Restricted diet, monitoring of blood sugar levels |
| **Leukemia**[§] | Weight loss, anorexia, pain in extremities, listlessness | Chemotherapy, intravenous fluids, transfusion(s) of blood and blood components, antibiotic therapy |

[§] Complication or comorbid condition

# Potassium (K)—
# Blood—Increased Level

**Reference Range: 3.5-5.0**

**Hospital Range:** _____

| Condition | Signs & Symptoms | Treatment |
|---|---|---|
| **Anemia, hemolytic** | Vomiting, anorexia, weight loss | Transfusion(s) of blood and blood components, chemotherapy, iron therapy, $O_2$ therapy |
| **Disease, Addison's[§]** | Features of crisis include anorexia, headache, weakness, dizziness, nausea, vomiting, apprehension, diarrhea, abdominal pain and syncope. Chronic Addison's disease may show indications resembling hypoglycemia (i.e., hunger, sweating, irritability, nervousness and depression). | Glucocorticoid and mineralocorticoid replacement |
| **Failure, renal, acute[§]** | Thirst, dyspnea, lethargy, weakness, anorexia, nausea | Management of diet, fluid and electrolytes; possible dialysis |
| **Hyperkalemia[§]** | Weakness and flaccid paralysis may occur. Often caused by renal insufficiency. | Diagnostic investigations to determine cause of hyperkalemia |

[§] Complication or comorbid condition

# Protein—
# Blood—Decreased Level

**Reference Range: 280-300**

**Hospital Range:** _____

| Condition | Signs & Symptoms | Treatment |
|-----------|------------------|-----------|
| **Burns** | Can result from thermal, electrical or chemical injuries. Severity is estimated by the size and depth of the burn. | Reverse isolation, skin grafts, intravenous fluids, invasive monitoring, high protein/high calorie diet |
| **Cirrhosis of liver**[§] | Abdominal pain or distention, fever, ascites, jaundice, anorexia | Sodium-restricted diet, intravenous fluids, treatment for relief of symptoms |
| **Hyper-natremia**[§] | Irritability, lethargy, weakness, confusion, stupor, coma | Intravenous fluids, force fluids, administration of $H_2O$ |
| **Malnutrition**[§] | Can be due to a number of diseases and can be a result of socioeconomic factors. Symptoms include muscle and fat wasting, edema, and electrolyte imbalances. | Nutritional therapy including oral dietary supplements and total parenteral nutrition (TPN) |

[§] Complication or comorbid condition

# Prothrombin Time—
# Increased Level

**Reference Range: 11-13 seconds
or 70-100%**

**Hospital Range:** _____

| Condition | Signs & Symptoms | Treatment |
|---|---|---|
| **Cirrhosis of liver**[§] | Abdominal pain or distention, fever, ascites, jaundice, anorexia | Sodium-restricted diet, intravenous fluids, treatment for relief of symptoms |
| **Disseminated intravascular coagulation (DIC)**[§] | Occurs as a complication of other conditions such as infection, neoplastic disease, burns, and obstetric complications. Characterized by abnormal bleeding such as from the gastrointestinal tract and small wounds such as intravenous sites. Bruising is also present. | Transfusion of plasma or platelets; intravenous heparin administration; intake and output monitoring |
| **Failure, heart, congestive**[§†‡] | Peripheral edema, shortness of breath. Cyanosis is present on occasion. Heart rate is irregular, moist rales at base of lungs with productive cough. Confusion is usually present. | Sodium-restricted diet, digitalis regulation, $O_2$ therapy, diuretics |
| **Hemophilia**[§] | Symptoms range from asymptomatic to severe bleeding as a result of minor trauma. Bleeding into joints and muscles can occur, with resultant swelling and pain. | Nonaspirin oral analgesia for pain. Deficient factor replacement required prior to even minor surgical procedures. |

[§] Complication or comorbid condition
[†] Cardiovascular complication
[‡] Complex diagnosis

# Reticulocyte Count—
# Decreased Level

**Reference Range: 0.5-1.5**

**Hospital Range:** _____

| Condition | Signs & Symptoms | Treatment |
|---|---|---|
| **Anemia, aplastic**[§] | Weakness, fatigue, shortness of breath | Reverse isolation, transfusion(s) of blood and blood components |
| **Anemia, hemolytic** | Vomiting, anorexia, weight loss | Transfusion(s) of blood and blood components, chemotherapy, iron therapy, $O_2$ therapy |
| **Anemia, hypochromic** | Tingling of extremities, dyspnea | Iron therapy, transfusion(s) of blood and blood components, $O_2$ therapy |
| **Cirrhosis of liver**[§] | Abdominal pain or distention, fever, ascites, jaundice, anorexia | Sodium-restricted diet, intravenous fluids, treatment for relief of symptoms |

[§] Complication or comorbid condition

# Reticulocyte Count—
# Increased Level

**Reference Range: 0.5-1.5**

**Hospital Range:** _____

| Condition | Signs & Symptoms | Treatment |
|---|---|---|
| **Anemia, aplastic** [§] | Weakness, fatigue, short-ness of breath | Reverse isolation, transfu-sion(s) of blood and blood components |
| **Anemia, hemolytic** | Vomiting, anorexia, weight loss | Transfusion(s) of blood and blood components, chemo-therapy, iron therapy, $O_2$ therapy |
| **Hemorrhage, not otherwise specified**[§] | Pallor, rapid shallow respirations, unstable vital signs, melena, hemoptysis, weakness, hematemesis | Intravenous therapy, trans-fusion(s) of blood and blood components, vitamin K, iron therapy |

[§] Complication or comorbid condition

# Sedimentation Rate—
# Increased Level

**Reference Range: Male 0-15**
**Female 0-25**

**Hospital Range:** _____

| Condition | Signs & Symptoms | Treatment |
|---|---|---|
| **Cancer of stomach**[§] | Weakness, constipation, abdominal pain, anorexia, weight loss, hematemesis, melena | Chemotherapy, radiation therapy, surgery, pain medications |
| **Endocarditis, bacterial** [§‡] | Skin lesions, weight loss, weakness, sweating, fever, heart murmur | Intravenous fluids, antibiotic therapy |
| **Infarction, acute myocardial** [§†] | Severe chest pain, gallop rhythm and other cardiac arrhythmias, shortness of breath, diaphoresis | Continuous monitoring, $O_2$ therapy, pain medication, intravenous fluids, intravenous medications, possible resuscitation |
| **Infections (acute)** | Fever, malaise, chills | Intravenous fluids, antibiotic therapy |

[§] Complication or comorbid condition
[‡] Complex diagnosis

# Serum Glutamic-Oxaloacetic Transminase (SGOT)— Increased Level

**Reference Range: 5-40**

**Hospital Range:** _____

| Condition | Signs & Symptoms | Treatment |
|---|---|---|
| **Cirrhosis of liver**[§] | Abdominal pain or distention, fever, ascites, jaundice, anorexia | Sodium-restricted diet, intravenous fluids, treatment for relief of symptoms |
| **Embolism, pulmonary**[§†‡] | Dyspnea, rales in lungs, sudden onset of substernal pain, dizziness, pallor | Heparin, diuretics |
| **Failure, heart, congestive**[§†‡] | Peripheral edema, shortness of breath. Cyanosis is present on occasion. Heart rate is irregular, moist rales at base of lungs with productive cough. Confusion is usually present. | Sodium-restricted diet, digitalis regulation, $O_2$ therapy, diuretics |
| **Infarction, myocardial, acute**[§] | Severe chest pain, gallop rhythm and other cardiac arrhythmias, shortness of breath, diaphoresis | Continuous monitoring, $O_2$ therapy, pain medication, intravenous fluids, intravenous medications, possible resuscitation |

[§] Complication or comorbid condition
[†] Cardiovascular complication
[‡] Complex diagnosis

# Serum Glutamic-Pyruvic Transminase—(SGPT) (ALT)—Increased Level

**Reference Range: 3-35**

**Hospital Range:** _____

| Condition | Signs & Symptoms | Treatment |
|-----------|------------------|-----------|
| **Infarction, myocardial, acute**[§] | Severe chest pain, gallop rhythm and other cardiac arrhythmias, shortness of breath, diaphoresis | Continuous monitoring, $O_2$ therapy, pain medication, intravenous medications, possible resuscitation |
| **Cirrhosis of liver**[§] | Abdominal pain or distention, fever, ascites, jaundice, anorexia | Sodium-restricted diet, intravenous fluids, treatment for relief of symptoms |
| **Failure, heart, congestive**[§†‡] | Peripheral edema, shortness of breath. Cyanosis is present on occasion. Heart rate is irregular, moist rales at base of lungs with productive cough. Confusion is usually present. | Sodium-restricted diet, digitalis regulation, $O_2$ therapy, diuretics |

[§] Complication or comorbid condition

[†] Cardiovascular complication

[‡] Complex diagnosis

# Sodium (Na)—
## Blood, Electrolytes—Decreased Level

**Reference Range: 135-145**

**Hospital Range: _____**

| Condition | Signs & Symptoms | Treatment |
|---|---|---|
| **Cirrhosis of liver**[§] | Abdominal pain or distention, fever, ascites, jaundice, anorexia | Sodium-restricted diet, intravenous fluids, treatment for relief of symptoms |
| **Disease, Addison's**[§] | Features of crisis include anorexia, headache, weakness, dizziness, nausea, vomiting, apprehension, diarrhea, abdominal pain and syncope. Chronic Addison's disease may show indications resembling hypoglycemia (i.e., hunger, sweating, irritability, nervousness and depression). | Glucocorticoid and mineralocorticoid replacement |
| **Failure, renal, chronic**[§] | Thirst, dyspnea, lethargy, weakness, anorexia, nausea, polyuria | Fluid restrictions, dialysis, transfusion(s) of blood and blood components |
| **Hyponatremia**[§] | Weakness, muscle cramps and spasms, confusion, irritability | Intravenous fluids, sodium concentrate |
| **Ketoacidosis**[§] | Irritability, weakness, excessive thirst, polyuria | Restricted diet, monitoring of blood sugar levels |

[§] Complication or comorbid condition

# Sodium (Na)—
# Blood, Electrolytes—Increased Level

**Reference Range: 135-145**

**Hospital Range:** _____

| Condition | Signs & Symptoms | Treatment |
|---|---|---|
| **Dehydration**[§] | Confusion, weakness, poor skin turgor, dry mucous membranes | Monitoring of electrolyte levels, intravenous therapy, force fluids, intake and output monitoring |
| **Failure, heart, congestive**[§†‡] | Peripheral edema, shortness of breath. Cyanosis is present on occasion. Heart rate is irregular, moist rales at base of lungs with productive cough. Confusion is usually present. | Sodium-restricted diet, digitalis regulation, $O_2$ therapy, diuretics |
| **Failure, renal, acute**[§] | Thirst, dyspnea, lethargy, weakness, anorexia, nausea | Management of diet, fluid and electrolytes; possible dialysis |
| **Hyper-natremia**[§] | Poor skin turgor, dry mucous membranes, confusion, stupor, coma | Intravenous fluids, force fluids, administration of $H_2O$ |

[§] Complication or comorbid condition

[†] Cardiovascular complication

[‡] Complex diagnosis

# Sodium (Na)—
# Urine—Decreased Level

**Reference Range: 40-220**

**Hospital Range:** _____

| Condition | Signs & Symptoms | Treatment |
|---|---|---|
| **Failure, heart, congestive**[§†‡] | Peripheral edema, shortness of breath. Cyanosis is present on occasion. Heart rate is irregular, moist rales at base of lungs with productive cough. Confusion is usually present. | Sodium-restricted diet, digitalis regulation, $O_2$ therapy, diuretics |
| **Failure, renal, chronic**[§] | Thirst, dyspnea, lethargy, weakness, anorexia, nausea, polyuria | Fluid restrictions, dialysis, transfusion(s) of blood and blood components |

[§] Complication or comorbid condition

[†] Cardiovascular complication

[‡] Complex diagnosis

# Sodium (Na)—
# Urine—Increased Level

## Reference Range: 40-220

**Hospital Range:** _____

| Condition | Signs & Symptoms | Treatment |
|---|---|---|
| **Disease, Addison's**[§] | Features of crisis include anorexia, headache, weakness, dizziness, nausea, vomiting, apprehension, diarrhea, abdominal pain and syncope. Chronic Addison's disease may show indications resembling hypoglycemia (i.e., hunger, sweating, irritability, nervousness and depression). | Glucocorticoid and mineralocorticoid replacement |
| **Dehydration**[§] | Confusion, weakness, poor skin turgor, dry mucous membranes | Monitoring of electrolyte levels, intravenous therapy, force fluids, intake and output monitoring |

[§] Complication or comorbid condition

# Total Iron Binding Capacity (TIBC)—
# Decreased Level

**Reference Range: 220-370**

**Hospital Range:** _____

| Condition | Signs & Symptoms | Treatment |
|---|---|---|
| **Anemia, aplastic**[§] | Weakness, fatigue, short-ness of breath | Reverse isolation, transfu-sion(s) of blood and blood components |
| **Anemia, sickle cell**[§] | Enlarged heart, tachy-cardia, heart murmurs, fatigue, dyspnea, joint and bone pain | Supportive care such as rest, analgesics, warm compresses. Transfusion of packed red blood cells may be necessary |
| **Cirrhosis of liver**[§] | Abdominal pain or distention, fever, ascites, jaundice, anorexia | Sodium-restricted diet, intravenous fluids, treat-ment for relief of symptoms |
| **Failure, renal, chronic**[§] | Weakness, bruising, dyspnea, lethargy, anor-exia, polyuria | Fluid restriction, dialysis, transfusion(s) of blood and blood components |
| **Infections (chronic)** | Symptoms vary with area of localization of infec-tion. Can include fever, nausea, vomiting. | Antibiotics, culture and sensitivity studies including blood cultures |

[§] Complication or comorbid condition

# TIBC—
# Increased Level

**Reference Range: 220-370**

**Hospital Range:** _____

| Condition | Signs & Symptoms | Treatment |
|---|---|---|
| **Anemia, hypo-chromic** | Tingling of extremities, dyspnea | Iron therapy, transfusion(s) of blood and blood components, $O_2$ therapy |
| **Anemia, iron deficiency** | Exertional dyspnea, fatigue, tachycardia | Iron supplements administered orally or parenterally |
| **Loss, blood acute/ chronic**[§] | Weakness, lethargy, shortness of breath pain | Intravenous fluids, transfusion(s) of blood and blood components, iron therapy |
| **Polycythemia vera** | Fatigue, pruritis, vertigo, dizziness, CVA, TIA | Phlebotomy, radiophosphorus (32P) |

[§] Complication or comorbid condition

# Uric Acid—
# Blood—Decreased Level

**Reference Range: 3-7**

**Hospital Range:** _____

| Condition | Signs & Symptoms | Treatment |
|-----------|------------------|-----------|
| **Burns** | Can result from thermal, electrical or chemical injuries. Severity is estimated by the size and depth of the burn. | Reverse isolation, skin graphs, intravenous fluids, invasive monitoring, high protein/high calorie diet |
| **Cirrhosis of liver**[§] | Abdominal pain or distention, fever, ascites, jaundice, anorexia | Sodium-restricted diet, intravenous fluids, treatment for relief of symptoms |

[§] Complication or comorbid condition

# Uric Acid—
## Blood—Increased Level

**Reference Range: 3-7**

**Hospital Range:** _____

| Condition | Signs & Symptoms | Treatment |
|---|---|---|
| **Cirrhosis of liver**[§] | Abnormal pain or distention, fever, ascites, jaundice, anorexia | Sodium-restricted diet, intravenous fluids, treatment for relief of symptoms |
| **Failure, renal, acute**[§] | Thirst, dyspnea, lethargy, fatigue, anorexia, nausea | Management of diet, fluid and electrolytes. Possible dialysis |
| **Gout** | Severe pain in joints, most usually affecting the metatarsophalangeal (MTP) joint | Colchicine, nonsteroidal antiinflammatory drugs, sometimes glucocorticoids, low protein diet |
| **Infarction, myocardial, acute**[§] | Severe chest pain, gallop rhythm and other cardiac arrhythmias, shortness of breath, diaphoresis | Continuous monitoring, $O_2$ therapy, pain medication, intravenous fluids, intravenous medications, possible resuscitation |
| **Leukemia, myelogenous, chronic**[§] | Anorexia, weight loss, weakness, fatigue, bruising, epistaxis, low-grade fever | Chemotherapy is primary treatment. Other treatments may include allopurinol to prevent increased uric acid and antibiotics for infections. |

[§] Complication or comorbid condition

# Urinalysis—
# Bile—Increased Level

**Reference Range: Negative**

**Hospital Range:** _____

| Condition | Signs & Symptoms | Treatment |
|---|---|---|
| **Calculus of bile duct**[§] | Epigastric pain and nausea, vomiting, jaundice | Intravenous fluids and medications, surgery |
| **Cirrhosis of liver**[§] | Abdominal pain or distention, fever, ascites, jaundice, anorexia | Sodium restricted diet, intravenous fluids, treatment for relief of symptoms |
| **Hepatitis**[§] | Jaundice, anorexia, dark urine, pruritis, light-colored stools | Rest, force fluids, anti-emetics for nausea, isolation precautions for blood and other body fluids |

[§] Complication or comorbid condition

# Urinalysis—
## Ketones or Acetones—Increased Level

**Reference Range: Negative**

**Hospital Range:** _____

| Condition | Signs & Symptoms | Treatment |
|---|---|---|
| **Ketoacidosis**[§] | Excessive thirst, poly-uria, irritability, weakness | Restricted diet, monitoring of blood sugar levels |
| **Ketosis, alco-holic**[§] | Vomiting and dehydra-tion in association with other symptoms of alcoholism such as DTs and cirrhosis | Intravenous infusion of normal saline and glucose |

[§] Complication or comorbid condition

# Urinalysis—
# pH—Decreased Level

**Reference Range: 4.5-8**

**Hospital Range:** _____

| Condition | Signs & Symptoms | Treatment |
|---|---|---|
| **Acidosis, metabolic**[§] | Hypotension, weakness, pallor, pulmonary edema | Fluid balance, electrolyte monitoring |
| **Acidosis, respiratory**[§] | Retention of $CO_2$ and increasing $pCO_2$; hypoventilation, dyspnea, drowsiness, weakness, malaise, nausea | Establishment of airway, $O_2$ therapy, artificial ventilation |
| **Dehydration**[§] | Confusion, weakness, poor skin turgor, dry mucous membranes | Monitoring of electrolyte levels, intravenous therapy, force fluids, intake and output monitoring |

[§] Complication or comorbid condition

# Urinalysis—
# pH—Increased Level

**Reference Range:** 4.6-8

**Hospital Range:** _____

| Condition | Signs & Symptoms | Treatment |
|---|---|---|
| **Failure, renal, chronic**[§] | Bruising, dyspnea, lethargy, weakness, anorexia, polyuria | Fluid restrictions, dialysis, transfusion(s) of blood and blood components |
| **Infection, urinary tract** [§] | Fever, dysuria, frequency, burning on urination | Urinary antiseptics, antibiotic therapy, intravenous fluids, force fluids |
| **Overdose, salicylate** | Tinnitus, diaphoresis, nausea, hyperventilation | Gastric lavage, activated charcoal, alkaline diuresis, may require dialysis |

[§] Complication or comorbid condition

# Urinalysis—
## Protein (Albumin)—Increased Level

**Reference Range: Negative**

**Hospital Range:** _____

| Condition | Signs & Symptoms | Treatment |
|---|---|---|
| **Disease, renal (glomerular, tubular, interstitial)**[§†] | Fatigue, vomiting, anorexia, polyuria | Fluid restrictions, dialysis |
| **Hematuria**[§] | Blood in the urine | Treatment of underlying cause (i.e., infection or trauma) |
| **Infection, urinary tract** [§] | Fever, dysuria, frequency, burning on urination | Urinary antiseptics, antibiotic therapy, intravenous fluids, force fluids |
| **Toxemia of pregnancy**[§] | Develops in the late second trimester or third trimester of pregnancy. Symptoms include hypertension, edema and weight gain.  In severe eclampsia, seizures and coma can occur. | Sedatives, bed rest, frequent monitoring of blood pressure, intake and output, daily weight. Cesarean section or induction of labor may be necessary. |

[§] Complication or comorbid condition
[†] Cardiovascular complication

# Urinalysis—
## Specific Gravity—Decreased Level

**Reference Range: 1.005-1.030**

**Hospital Range:** _____

| Condition | Signs & Symptoms | Treatment |
|-----------|------------------|-----------|
| **Disease, renal (glomerular, tubular, interstitial)**[§†] | Fatigue, vomiting, anorexia, polyuria | Fluid restrictions, dialysis |
| **Hypokalemia** | Nausea and vomiting, anorexia | Potassium supplement, intravenous fluid |

[§] Complication or comorbid condition
[†] Cardiovascular complication

# Urinalysis—
## Specific Gravity—Increased Level

**Reference Range: 1.005-1.030**

**Hospital Range:** _____

| Condition | Signs & Symptoms | Treatment |
|---|---|---|
| **Dehydration**[§] | Confusion, weakness, poor skin turgor, dry mucous membranes | Monitoring of electrolyte levels, intravenous therapy, force fluids, intake and output monitoring |
| **Failure, heart, congestive**[§†‡] | Peripheral edema, shortness of breath. Cyanosis is present on occasion. Heart rate is irregular, moist rales at base of lungs with productive cough. Confusion is usually present. | Sodium-restricted diet, digitalis regulation, $O_2$ therapy, diuretics |

[§] Complication or comorbid condition
[†] Cardiovascular complication
[‡] Complex diagnosis

# Urinalysis—
## Urobilinogen—Increased Level

**Reference Range: <0.1**

**Hospital Range:** _____

| Condition | Signs & Symptoms | Treatment |
|-----------|------------------|-----------|
| **Anemia, hemolytic** | Vomiting, anorexia, weight loss | Transfusion(s) of blood and blood components, chemotherapy, iron therapy, $O_2$ therapy |
| **Cirrhosis of liver**[§] | Abdominal pain or distention, fever, ascites, jaundice, anorexia | Sodium-restricted diet, intravenous fluids, treatment for relief of symptoms |

[§] Complication or comorbid condition

# Urinalysis: Microscopic Exam—
# Cast Hyaline—Increased Level

**Reference Range: 0-4/lpf**

**Hospital Range:** _____

| Condition | Signs & Symptoms | Treatment |
|---|---|---|
| **Failure, heart, congestive**[§†‡] | Peripheral edema, shortness of breath. Cyanosis is present on occasion. Heart rate is irregular, moist rales at base of lungs with productive cough. Confusion is usually present. | Sodium-restricted diet, digitalis regulation, $O_2$ therapy, diuretics |
| **Disease, renal (glomerular, tubular, interstitial)**[§†] | Fatigue, vomiting, anorexia, polyuria | Fluid restrictions, dialysis |

[§] Complication or comorbid condition
[†] Cardiovascular complication
[‡] Complex diagnosis

# Urinalysis: Microscopic Exam—
# White Blood Cells (WBCs)—
# Increased Level

**Reference Range: 0-4/hpf**

**Hospital Range:** _____

| Condition | Signs & Symptoms | Treatment |
|---|---|---|
| **Pyelone-phritis**[§] | Fever, chills, flank pain, urinary frequency, dysuria | Antibiotic therapy, urinary analgesics, surgery if obstruction is present, force fluids |
| **Urinary tract infection**[§] | Fever, dysuria, frequency, burning on urination | Urinary antiseptics, antibiotic therapy, intravenous fluids, force fluids |

[§] Complication or comorbid condition

# Urine Culture—
# Presence of Pathogens

**Reference Range: Negative**

**Hospital Range:** _____

| Condition | Signs & Symptoms | Treatment |
|---|---|---|
| **Urinary tract infection**[§] | Fever, dysuria, frequency, burning on urination | Urinary antiseptics, antibiotic therapy, intravenous fluids, force fluids |

[§] Complication or comorbid condition

# Chapter 3: Organisms

| Specimen Site | Information to Look for |
|---|---|
| **Bladder** | *Normal Condition of Flora:* Specimen is normally sterile and free of organism growth.<br><br>*Possible Pathogens:* Any organism. Common contaminants are Enterobacter, Escherichia coli, Klebsiella and Staphylococcus epidermidis. |
| **Blood (multiple cultures usually performed)** | *Normal Condition of Flora:* Specimen is normally sterile and free of organism growth.<br><br>*Possible Pathogens:* Any organism. Common contaminant is Staphylococcus epidermidis. Most common pathogens are Bacteroides species, Haemophilus influenzae, Staphylococcus aureus and Streptococcus pyogenes. |
| **Body fluids: pleural, peritoneal, pericardial, synovial, seminal** | *Normal Condition of Flora:* Specimen is normally sterile and free of organism growth.<br><br>*Possible Pathogens:* Any organism. Common contaminant is Staphylococcus epidermidis. Pathogens include Bacteroides species, Escherichia coli and Neisseria gonorrhoeae. |
| **Cerebrospinal fluid** | *Normal Condition of Flora:* Specimen is normally sterile and free of organism growth.<br><br>*Possible Pathogens:* Any organism. Common contaminant is Staphylococcus epidermidis. Pathogens include Escherichia coli, Haemophilus influenzae, Neisseria meningitidis and Streptococci agalactiae. |
| **Cervix** | *Normal Condition of Flora:* Diphtheroids, Escherichia coli, Lactobacilli, nonhemolytic Streptococcus and Staphylococcus epidermidis.<br><br>*Possible Pathogens:* Candida albicans (in large numbers), Gardnerella vaginalis, Neisseria gonorrhoeae and Trichomonas. |

| Specimen Site | Information to Look for |
|---|---|
| **Duodenum** | *Normal Condition of Flora:* Enterococci and Lactobacilli.<br><br>*Possible Pathogens:* Giardia lamblia and Parasites. These organisms will not be grown on bacterial culture media. Recovered from examination for ova and parasites. |
| **Ear** | *Normal Condition of Flora:* Bacillus species, Diptheroids, Saprophytic fungi and Staphylococcus epidermis.<br><br>*Possible Pathogens:* Streptococcus pneumoniae is the most significant. Candida albicans, Haemophilus influenzae, Proteus species, Pseudomonas species and Staphylococcus aureus. |
| **Eye** | *Normal Condition of Flora:* Diptheroids, Moraxella species, Neisseria species and Staphylococcus epidermis.<br><br>*Possible Pathogens:* Any organisms. Common pathogens include Haemophilus influenzae, Staphylococcus aureus and Streptococcus viridans. |
| **Kidney** | *Normal Condition of Flora:* Specimen is normally sterile and free of organism growth.<br><br>*Possible Pathogens:* Any organism. Most common are Staphylococcus and Streptococci. |
| **Large intestine** | *Normal Condition of Flora:* Aspergillus, Bacillus subtilis, Bacteroides, Candida, Clostridium species, Diptheroids, Enterobacter, Enterococci, Escherichia coli, Fusobacterium, Klebsiella, Lactobacilli, Peptococcus, Peptostreptococcus, Proteus species, Pseudomonas species and Staphylococci.<br><br>*Possible Pathogens:* Campylobacter species, Candida albicans in large numbers, Salmonella species, Shigella species, Vibrio cholera and Yersinia species. |

| Specimen Site | Information to Look for |
|---|---|
| **Lower ileum** | *Normal Condition of Flora:* Clostridium perfringens, Enterococcus, occasionally Escherichia coli, Lactobacilli, Staphylococci, Streptococcus of viridans group.<br><br>*Possible Pathogens:* Salmonella species and Shigella species. |
| **Mouth** | *Normal Condition of Flora:* (After newborn period) Bacteroids, Branhamella catarrhalis, Candida albicans, Diphtheroids, Escherichia coli, Haemophilus species, Neisseria murosa, Peptostreptococcus lactobacillus, Staphylococcus epidermidis and Streptococcus of viridans group.<br><br>*Possible Pathogens:* Candida albicans in large numbers, Haemophilus influenzae and Haemophilus parainfluenzae, Staphylococcus aureus (in large numbers), Streptococcus Group A. |
| **Nasopharynx** | *Normal Condition of Flora:* (Sterile at birth) Bacteroids, Diphtheroids, Escherichia coli, gram positive bacilli, Haemophilus influenzae, Neisseria species, Staphylococci, Streptococci, Streptococcus pneumoniae and Proteus species.<br><br>*Possible Pathogens:* Bordetella pertussis, Corynebacterium diptheriae. In large numbers: Escherichia coli, gram negative bacilli, Haemophilus species, Proteus species, Pseudomonas species, Staphylococcus aureus and Streptococcus pneumoniae. |
| **Nose** | *Normal Condition of Flora:* Diphtheroids, Enterobacter species, gram positive bacilli, Klebsiella species, Staphylococcus species and Streptococcus species.<br><br>*Possible Pathogens:* Haemophilus influenzae, Staphylococcus aureus and Streptococcus pyogenes Group A. |

| Specimen Site | Information to Look for |
|---|---|
| **Skin** | *Normal Condition of Flora:* Acinetobacter, alpha-hemolytic Streptococci, Candida albicans, Diphtheroids, Enterococci, Enterococci Propioni-bacterium, Proteus, Staphylococcus epidermidis and Staphylococcus species.<br><br>*Possible Pathogens:* Clostridium species, Corynebacterium diphtheriae, Escherichia coli, Klebsiella, Neisseria-Staphylococcus aureus, Staphylococcus pyogenes. |
| **Sputum** | *Normal Condition of Flora:* Specimen normally free of organism growth.<br><br>*Possible Pathogens:* Any organism. Common contaminants are oral bacteria. The greater the number of squamous epithelial cells, the greater the contamination by oral-pharynx materials. Most common pathogens include gram negative bacilli or Staphylococcus aureus. Others are Haemophilus influenzae and Streptococcus pneumoniae. |
| **Stool, feces** | *Normal Condition of Flora:* Bacteroids, Clostridium albicans (in large numbers), Diphtheroids, Enterobacter species, Escherichia coli, Fusobacterium, Klebsiella species, Lactobacillus species, Peptococcus species, Peptostreptococcus species, Proteus species, Pseudomonas species, Staphylococcus species, Streptococcus species and yeast.<br><br>*Possible Pathogens:* Campylobacter species, Candida albicans (in large numbers), Salmonella species, Shigella species, Vibrio cholera and Yersenia species. Candida albicans can be pathogenic when preceded by antibiotic therapy. |
| **Throat** | *Normal Condition of Flora:* Diphtheroids, Escherichia coli, Haemophilus species, Staphylococcus species, Streptococcus species.<br><br>*Possible Pathogens:* Bordetella pertussis, Corynebacterium diptheriae, Haemophilus species. In large numbers: Escherichia coli, Proteus species, Pseudomonas species, Staphylococcus aureus, Streptococcus pneumoniae, Streptococcus pyogenes Group A. |

| Specimen Site | Information to Look for |
|---|---|
| **Trachea, bronchi, to lungs, sinus cavities** | *Normal Condition of Flora:* Specimen is normally sterile and free of organism growth.<br><br>*Possible Pathogens:* Candida albicans, Coccidioides, Escherichia coli or Proteus mirabilis, Haemophilus influenzae, Klebsiella, Mycoplasma pneumoniae, parainfluenza virus, Pneumocystis, Pseudomonas, Salmonella, Staphylococci, Streptococcus pneumoniae. |
| **Ureter** | *Normal Condition of Flora:* Specimen is normally sterile and free of organism growth.<br><br>*Possible Pathogens:* Any organism. Most common pathogen is Escherichia coli. Proteus, Pseudomonas and Staphylococcus aureus are others. |
| **Urethra** | *Normal Condition of Flora:* Diphtheroids and Enterococcus, Mycoplasma, Staphylococcus epidermidis.<br><br>*Possible Pathogens:* Candida albicans, Neisseria gonorrhoeae and Trichomonas. |
| **Urine, clean catch** | *Normal Condition of Flora:* Specimen is normally sterile and free of organism growth.<br><br>*Possible Pathogens:* Any organism count greater than 100,000 organisms per milliliter. Chronic infection may have repeatedly lower colony counts. Common contaminant is Staphylococcus epidermidis. Most common pathogen is Escherichia coli. Others include Proteus, Pseudomonas and Staphylococcus aureus. |
| **Vagina** | *Normal Condition of Flora:* (Adult) Candida albicans, Clostridium sporogenes, Diphtheroids, Escherichia coli, Lactobacilli, nonhemolytic and alphahemolytic Streptococcus species, Staphylococcus epidermidis and Yeasts.<br><br>*Possible Pathogens:* Candida albicans (in large numbers), Gardnerella vaginalis, Neisseria gonorrhoeae, and Trichomonas. |

| Specimen Site | Information to Look for |
|---|---|
| **Wound or abscess** | *Normal Condition of Flora:* Specimen is normally sterile and free of organism growth.<br><br>*Possible Pathogens:* Clostridium species, Escherichia coli, Pseudomonas species, Proteus species, Staphylococcus aureus, Streptococcus pyogenes Group A. Common contaminant is Staphylococcus epidermidis. |

# Chapter 4: Drug Usage

| Drug | Drug Action | Indications |
|------|-------------|-------------|
| **Adapin, Sinequan;** [doxepin hydrochloride] | Antidepressant | Used to relieve mild to severe symptoms of depression. |
| **Adriamycin** [doxorubicin hydrochloride] | Cytotoxic, antibiotic | Used to produce regression in disseminated neoplastic conditions, such as acute lymphoblastic leukemia and various types of carcinomas. |
| **Aldactazide, Aldactone** [spironolactone] | Diuretic, antihypertensive | Used for treatment of edematous conditions due to congestive heart failure, cirrhosis of liver, nephrotic syndrome and essential hypertension. |
| **Aldomet** [methyldopa] | Antihypertensive | Used for treatment of hypertension. |
| **Aldoril** [hydrochlorothiazide & methyldopa] | Antihypertensive, diuretic | Used for long-term treatment of moderate to severe hypertension, particularly in patients with edema and renal dysfunction. |
| **Alupent, Metaprel** [metaproterenol sulfate] | Bronchodilator | Indicated for use in treatment of bronchial asthma and for reversible bronchospasm in bronchitis and emphysema. |
| **Amicar** [aminocaproic acid] | Systemic hemostatic | Used in life-threatening situations to prevent clot dissolution. |
| **Amikin, Amikacin** [amikacin sulfate] | Aminoglycoside antibiotic | Active in treatment of gram-negative bacterial infections such as Pseudomonas, Escherichia coli, Proteus, Klebsiella-Enterobacter-Serratia. Therapeutic level: peak: 15-30 mcg/ml; trough: 5-10 mcg/ml. Toxic level: peak: > 35mcg/ml; trough: > 10mcg/ml. |

| Drug | Drug Action | Indications |
|---|---|---|
| **Aminophylline** [theophylline ethylenediamine] | Bronchodilator, pulmonary vasodilator, smooth muscle relaxant | Used for relief and/or prevention of symptoms from asthma and reversible bronchospasms in bronchitis and emphysema. Therapeutic level: 10-20 mcg/ml. Toxic level: > 20 mcg/ml. |
| **Amyl nitrite** | Vasodilator | Used as muscle relaxant that produces prompt, short-term relief of angina pectoris and renal or gallbladder colic. |
| **Amytal** [amobarbital sodium] | Sedative, hypnotic | Used for acute convulsive disorders. |
| **Ancef** | Semi-synthetic cephalosporin antibiotic | Respiratory tract infections due to streptococcus pneumoniae, klebsiella species, haeophilus infuenzae, staphylococcus aureus and group A beta-hemolytic streptocci. Urinary tract infections due to Eschericia coli, Proteus mirabiis, Klebsiella species and some stains of enterobacter and enterococci. Skin and skin structure infections, biliary tract infections, bone and joint infections, genital infections, septicemia, and endocarditis. |
| **Anectine** [succinylcholine chloride] | Depolarizing blocker | Used for muscle relaxation during surgery, endotracheal intubation, electroshock therapy, endoscopy and short manipulative procedures. |
| **Anginar** [erythrol tetranitrate] | Coronary vasodilator | Used for long-term management of angina rather than for short-term relief; has slower onset but sustained duration of action similar to nitroglycerin. |
| **Antabuse** [disulfiram] | Alcohol treatment | Used to treat alcoholism. |

| Drug | Drug Action | Indications |
|---|---|---|
| **Antivert** | Antihistamine | Management of nausea and vomiting, and dizziness associated with motion sickness. |
| **Apresoline** [hydralazine hydrochloride] | Antihypertensive | Used for management of essential hypertension. |
| **Aramine** [metaraminol bitartrate] | Adrenergic agent | Used for hypotension associated with surgery, anesthesia, hemorrhage, trauma, infections and adverse drug reactions. |
| **Arlidin** [nylidrin hydrochloride] | Beta-receptor stimulant | Used for treatment of vasospastic disorders such as peripheral vascular disease and circulatory disturbances of the inner ear. |
| **Ascriptin** [acetylsalicylic acid (ASA)] | Analgesic, antiinflammatory, antipyretic | Used for treatment of rheumatoid arthritis, osteoarthritis and other arthritic conditions. |
| **Atarax** [hydroxyzine hydrochloride] | Antianxiety agent, hypnotic | Used for relief of anxiety and tension, associated with psychoneurosis and as adjunct therapy in organic disease states in which anxiety is manifested. |
| **Ativan** [lorazepam] | Antianxiety agent, hypnotic | Used for controlling tension, anxiety, agitation, irritability and insomnia. |
| **Bactrim** [trimethoprim sulfamethoxazole] | Antibacterial | Used in treatment of urinary tract infections, acute otitis media, acute exacerbation of chronic bronchitis, shigellosis and pneumocystis carinii. |
| **Barbital** [barbital sodium] | Sedation, mild but prolonged | Used as long-acting sedative. |

| Drug | Drug Action | Indications |
|------|-------------|-------------|
| **Benadryl** [diphenhydramine hydrochloride] | Antihistamine, anticholinergic | Used for treatment of parkinsonism and allergies. |
| **Bentyl** [dicyclomine hydrochloride] | Antispasmodic | Used to treat hypermotility and spasms in gastrointestinal tract associated with irritable bowel, ulcerative colitis, diverticulitis and peptic ulcer disease. |
| **Betoptic** | Cardioselective beta-adrenergic receptor blocking agent | Lowers intraocular pressure and is also used for treatment of ocular hypertension and chronic open-angle glaucoma. |
| **Brethine** [terbutaline sulfate] | Bronchodilator | Used in management of bronchial asthma and reversible bronchospasm, and as tocolytic agent. |
| **Bronkosol** [isoetharine hydrochloride] | Bronchodilator | Used in management of bronchial asthma and reversible bronchospasm. |
| **Butazolidin** [phenylbutazone] | Antiinflammatory | Used to treat gout, spondylitis, psoriasis, rheumatoid arthritis, osteoarthritis and postoperative and posttraumatic inflammation. |
| **Butisol** [butabarbital sodium] | Hypnotic, mild sedative | Used more as a sedative than a hypnotic; used for patients with anxiety. |
| **Calan** (verapamil hydrochloride) | Antianginal preparation | Prescribed for angina at rest, including vasospastic and unstable angina, chronic stable angina, and control of ventricular rate. |

| Drug | Drug Action | Indications |
|------|-------------|-------------|
| **Cardilate** [erythrol tetranitrate] | Coronary vasodilator | Used for long-term management of angina rather than for short-term relief; has slower onset but sustained duration of action similar to nitroglycerin. |
| **Catapres** [clonidine hydrochloride] | Antihypertensive | Used for mild to moderate hypertension; sometimes used for migraine, menopausal flushing or dysmenorrhea therapy. |
| **Clinoril** [sulindac] | Antiinflammatory | Used for treatment of osteoarthritis, rheumatoid arthritis, ankylosing spondylitis and gouty arthritis. |
| **Clomid** [clomiphene citrate] | Ovarian stimulant | Used to treat female infertility. |
| **Clonopin** [clonazepam] | Anticonvulsant | Used for petit mal epilepsy or akinetic and myoclonic seizures. |
| **Cogentin** (Benztropine Mesylate) | Antiparkinsonism | Used to treat Parkinson's disease. |
| **Colace** [dioctyl sodium sulfosuccinate] | Stool softener | Used in treatment of constipation, painful anorectal conditions, cardiac and other conditions in which maximum ease of passage is desirable. |
| **Colestid** [colestipol hydrochloride] | Antihyperlipidemic | Used for hypercholesterolemia therapy. |
| **Compazine** [prochlorperazine] | Antiemetic, antipsychotic | Used to treat nausea, vomiting and manic phase of bipolar syndrome. |
| **Coumadin** [sodium warfarin] | Thrombolytic agent | Used in prophylaxis and treatment of venous thrombosis, treatment of atrial fibrillation with embolization (pulmonary embolism). |

| Drug | Drug Action | Indications |
|------|-------------|-------------|
| **Cycols-pasmol** [cyclandelate] | Peripheral vasodilator | Used for mild peripheral dilation by relaxing smooth spasmolytic muscles. |
| **Cytomel** | Thyroid hormone | Used for treatment of hypothyroidism or prevention of euthyroid goiters. |
| **Dalmane** [flurazepam] | Hypnotic, antianxiety agent | Used as a sleeping aid. |
| **Darvon-N** [propoxyphe ne napsylate] | Analgesic | Used to relieve mild to moderate pain and to suppress withdrawal symptoms from narcotics. |
| **Daypro** (oxaprozin) | Nonsteroidal antiinflamma-tory drug (NSAID) | Indicated for management of osteoar-thritis and rheumatoid arthritis. |
| **Dextran-75** | Blood volume expander | Used for shock, severe hemorrhage and cardiovascular surgery. |
| **Diabinese** [chlorpropa-mide] | Antidiabetic | Used as adjunct to diet in noninsulin-dependent diabetes mellitus (type II). |
| **Dilaudid** [hydromor-phone hydro-chloride] | Narcotic anal-gesic | Used as analgesic for severe pain, as pre- and post-operative medication; used for terminally ill patients. |
| **Didronel** [etidronate disodium] | Bone-growth regulator | Used for Paget's disease and hetero-topic ossification due to spinal cord injury. |
| **Diflucan** (Fluconazole) | Antifungal agent | Used in oropharyngeal and esophageal candidiasis and cryptococcal meningitis in AIDS patients. |
| **Digitalis** | Cardiotonic glycoside | Used in treatment of heart failure, atrial flutter, atrial fibrillation and supraven-tricular tachycardia. |

| Drug | Drug Action | Indications |
|------|-------------|-------------|
| **Dilantin** [phenytoin sodium] | Anticonvulsant | Used for control of grand mal and psychomotor seizures. Therapeutic level: 10-20 mcg/ml. Toxic level: > 30 mcg/ml. |
| **D-Mannitol** [mannitol] | Diuretic, osmotic | Used to promote fluid loss, especially when renal impairment exists. |
| **Dulcolax** [bisacodyl] | Cathartic, stimulant | Used to clean colon in preparation for diagnostic procedures or following such procedures; used for chronic constipation or with colostomies. |
| **Dymelor** [acetohexamide] | Oral antidiabetic | Used to treat newly diagnosed to moderately severe diabetes. |
| **Elavil, Endep** [amitriptyline hydrochloride] | Antidepressant | Used as sedative or antidepressant. |
| **Emete-Con** [benzquinamide hydrochloride] | Antiemetic | Used to prevent and treat nausea during anesthesia and surgery. |
| **Epinephrine** [adrenaline hydrochloride] | Bronchodilator, cardiotonic | Most commonly used to relieve respiratory distress due to bronchospasm and to restore cardiac rhythm in cardiac arrest. |
| **Ergomar** [ergotamine tartrate] | Alphaadrenergic | Used as drug of choice for migraine or cluster headache therapy. |
| **Ergotrate** [ergonovine maleate] | Oxytocic agent | Used to prevent postpartal hemorrhage and occasionally to treat migraine headaches. |
| **Estrace** [estradiol] | Estrogen therapy | Used to treat menopausal symptoms, functional uterine bleeding, amenorrhea, inoperable prostatic cancer and postpartum breast engorgement. |

| Drug | Drug Action | Indications |
|------|-------------|-------------|
| **Flexeril** [cyclobenza-prine hydro-chloride] | Muscle relaxant | Used as adjunct to rest and physical therapy for muscle spasms. |
| **Follutein** [chorionic gonadot-ropin] | Gonadot-ropic hormone | Used for prepubital cryptorchidism, hypogonadism, corpus luteum insufficiency and infertility. |
| **Glucotrol** (glipizide) | Oral blood-glucose-lowering agent | Used an an adjunct to diet for the control of hyperglycemia in patients with noninsulin dependent diabetes mellitus (NIDDM; type II). |
| **Haldol** [halo-peridol] | Antipsychotic | Used for treatment of Tourette's syndrome, acute and chronic psychoses and psychotic reactions in adults with brain damage and mental retardation. |
| **Heparin** [heparin sodium] | Anticoagulant | Used for prophylaxis and treatment of venous thrombosis, pulmonary embolism, prevention of cerebral thrombosis and treatment of consumptive coagulopathies. |
| **Hydergine** [ergot alkaloids dihydrogenated] | Antiadrenergic | Used for idiopathic decline in mental capacity. |
| **HydroDIURIL** [hydrochlorothiazide] | Diuretic, anti-hypertensive | Used in management of hypertension and in adjunctive therapy for edema associated with congestive heart failure, hepatic cirrhosis, corticosteroid and estrogen therapy. |
| **Hyperstat IV** [diazoxide] | Antihypertensive | Used for hypertensive crisis, especially in patients with renal impairment, eclampsia, left ventricular hypertrophy or hypertensive encephalopathy. |
| **Hytuss** [guaifenesin] | Expectorant | Used to treat symptoms of productive cough. |

| Drug | Drug Action | Indications |
|------|-------------|-------------|
| **Imferon** [iron dextran] | Antianemic | Injectable used for iron-deficient patients suffering from anemias. |
| **Imodium** [loperamide hydrochloride] | Antidiarrheal | Used to relieve acute, nonspecific diarrhea. |
| **Inapsine** [droperidol] | Antipsychotic, antianxiety agent | Used preoperatively and as adjunctive therapy to anesthesia. |
| **Inderal** [propranolol hydrochloride] | Beta-adrenergic blocking agent | Used for management of hypertension, long-term management of angina pectoris due to coronary atherosclerosis, cardiac arrhythmias. |
| **Indocin** [indomethacin] | Antiinflammatory antipyretic | Used for acute and moderate rheumatoid arthritis and osteoarthritis and as an antipyretic in Hodgkin's disease. |
| **INH** [isoniazid] | Tuberculosis preparation | Used for treatment of all forms of tuberculosis in which organisms are susceptible. |
| **Innovar** [fentanyl and droperidol] | Narcotic analgesic, antipsychotic | Used to produce tranquilization and analgesia for surgical or diagnostic procedures; may be used for anesthetic premedication. |
| **Intropin** [dopamine hydrochloride] | Inotropic agent | Used for correction of hemodynamic imbalances present in shock syndrome due to acute myocardial infarction, andotoxic septicemia, open heart surgery, renal failure and chronic cardiac decompensation. |
| **Isordil** [isosorbide dinitrate] | Smooth muscle relaxant | Used for treatment of acute anginal attacks. |

| Drug | Drug Action | Indications |
|------|-------------|-------------|
| **Isuprel** [isoproterenol sulfate] | Adrenergic agent | Used as bronchodilator for asthma, chronic pulmonary emphysema, bronchitis and other conditions accompanied by bronchoopaom; oan bo uood in cardiogenic shock cases. |
| **Kefzol** [cefazolin sodium] | Antibiotic | Used in treatment of serious infections such as respiratory tract, genitourinary tract, skin and soft tissue, biliary tract infections, septicemia and endocarditis. |
| **Ketochol** [ketocholanic acid] | Digestant | Used as a laxative. |
| **K-Lyte** [potassium chloride] | Potassium supplement | Used in therapy of prophylaxis of potassium deficiency. |
| **Lanoxin** [digoxin] | Cardiotonic | Used in the treatment of congestive heart failure. Therapeutic level: 0.9-2 ng/ml. Toxic level: > 2 ng/ml. |
| **Lasix** [furosemide] | Diuretic | Used for management of edema associated with congestive heart failure, renal disease, including the nephrotic syndrome and hypertension. |
| **L-dopa** [levodopa] | Antiparkinsonian | Used to treat Parkinson's disease. |
| **Levo-Dromoran** [levorphanol tartrate] | Narcotic analgesic | Used as analgesia for severe pain, as pre- and postoperative medication. |
| **Levsin** [hyoscyamine sulfate] | Belladonna alkaloid | Used in antispasmodic and anticholinergic therapy. |
| **Librium** [chlordiazepoxide] | Antianxiety agent | Used for patients with acute withdrawal symptoms, especially from alcohol, or for other anxiety-producing conditions. |

| Drug | Drug Action | Indications |
|------|-------------|-------------|
| **Lidocaine** [lidocaine hydrochloride] | Antiarrhythmic | Used for management of ventricular arrhythmias or during cardiac manipulation, such as cardiac surgery. Therapeutic level: 2-5 mcg/ml. Toxic level: > 6 mcg/ml. |
| **Lithium** | Antipsychotic | Used to control manic episodes in bipolar syndrome. |
| **Lomotil** [diphenoxylate hydrochloride with atropine] | Antidiarrheal | Used to treat symptoms of chronic and functional diarrhea. |
| **Lopressor** [metoprolol tartrate] | Antihypertensive, beta-blocker | Used for hypertension therapy. |
| **Lorelco** [probucol] | Antihyperlipidemic | Used for hyperlipoproteinemia. |
| **Lorfan** [levallorphan tartrate] | Narcotic antagonist | Used to overcome respiratory de-pression induced by drug overdose. |
| **Mandol** [cefamandole nafate] | Antibiotic | Used for treatment of lower respiratory infections, urinary tract infections, peritonitis, septicemia. |
| **Megace** [megestrol acetate] | Progestin, synthetic | Used in palliative treatment of endometrial or breast cancer. |
| **Mellaril** [thioridazine hydrochloride] | Antipsychotic | Used to treat acute and chronic schizophrenia and hyperactivity (in children). |
| **Meprospan or Miltown** [meprobamate] | Antianxiety agent | Used for simple insomnia and as premedication for electroshock therapy and muscle relaxant therapy. |

| Drug | Drug Action | Indications |
|------|-------------|-------------|
| **Methergine** [methyler-gonovine maleate] | Oxytocic agent | Used for routine management of post-partum hemorrhage after delivery of placenta. |
| **Micro-K** [potassium chloride] | Potassium supplement | Used therapeutically for hypokalemia or digitalis intoxication. |
| **Milk of Magnesia** [magnesium carbonate] | Antacid, laxative | Used as antacid or laxative. |
| **Minipress** [prazosin hydrochloride] | Antihypertensive | Used for mild to moderate hypertension. |
| **Mucomyst** [acetylcysteine] | Expectorant | Used for acute and chronic bronchitis, emphysema and other bronchopulmonary disorders. |
| **Myambutol** [ethambutol hydrochloride] | Oral chemotherapeutic agent | Used for treatment of pulmonary tuberculosis. |
| **Mylanta** [aluminum magnesium & simethicone] | Antacid, antiflatulent | Used for relief of symptoms associated with gastric hyperacidity and flatus (trapped gas). |
| **Mysoline** [primidone] | Anticonvulsant | Used for psychomotor seizures, myoclonic epilepsy or refractory grand mal epilepsy. |
| **Nalfon** [fenoprofen calcium] | Antiinflammatory | Used for rheumatoid arthritis and osteoarthritis. |
| **Naprosyn** [naproxen] | Antiinflammatory | Used for rheumatoid arthritis and osteoarthritis. |

| Drug | Drug Action | Indications |
|------|-------------|-------------|
| **Narcan** [naloxone hydrochloride] | Narcotic antagonist | Used to reverse respiratory depression induced by narcotics overdose. |
| **Navane** [thiothixene] | Antipsychotic | Used to treat symptoms of acute and chronic schizophrenia. |
| **Nembutal** [pentobarbital sodium] | Sedative, hypnotic | Used as adjunct medication in diagnostic procedures or for emergency use with convulsive disorders. |
| **Niacin** [nicotinic acid] | Anticholesterol agent | Used to reduce blood cholesterol, blood fatty acids and lipids. |
| **Nipride** [sodium nitroprusside] | Antihypertensive | Used for potent, rapid action in reducing blood pressure in hypertensive crisis or for controlling bleeding during anesthesia by producing controlled hypotension. |
| **Nitroglycerin** [glyceryl trinitrate] | Muscle relaxant | Used for prophylaxis and treatment of angina pectoris. |
| **Noctec** [chloral hydrate] | Nonbarbiturate sedative, hypnotic | Used as general hypnotic or sedative; used for patients undergoing chemical withdrawal. |
| **Norflex** [orphenadrine citrate] | Muscle relaxant | Used for acute spasms, tension and posttrauma cases. |
| **Norpace** [disopyramide] | Antiarrhythmic | Used for coronary artery disease, for prevention, recurrence and control of unifocal, multifocal and paired PVCs. |
| **Norvasc** (amlodipine besylate) | Calcium channel blocker | Used in hypertension, chronic stable angina and vasospastic angina. |
| **Orinase** [tobutamide sodium] | Oral antidiabetic | Used for oral diabetic therapy. |

| Drug | Drug Action | Indications |
|------|-------------|-------------|
| **Panteric** [pancreatin] | Digestant | Used for pancreatic enzyme deficiency; used for invalids with poor digestion. |
| **Paral** [paraldehyde] | Sedative, hypnotic | Used for sleep induction. |
| **Pavabid** [papaverine hydrochloride] | Cerebral, vasodilator | Used for relief of cerebral and peripheral ischemia. |
| **Pavulon** [pancuronium bromide] | Competitive blocker | Used for muscle relaxation during surgery and endotracheal intubation. |
| **Percodan** [oxycodone terephthalate] | Narcotic analgesic | Used for moderate acute pain relief for bursitis, injuries, dislocations, simple fractures, postpartum conditions, neuralgia, etc. |
| **Pergonal** [menotropins] | Ovarian stimulant | Used for infertility caused by secondary ovarian failure and primary or secondary amenorrhea. |
| **Persantine** [dipyridamole] | Coronary vasodilator | Therapy for chronic angina pectoris. |
| **Phenacetin** [acetophenetidin] | Analgesic, antiinflammatory | Used to control fever, pain, myalgia, headache and dysmenorrhea. |
| **Phenobarbital** | Sedative, anticonvulsant, antiepileptic | Used for grand mal epilepsy. |
| **Pitocin** [oxytocin citrate] | Oxytocic agent | Used to induce or stimulate labor at term. |

| Drug | Drug Action | Indications |
|------|-------------|-------------|
| **Plasmanate** [plasma, plasma protein fraction] | Blood volume expander | Used for hypovolemic shock, burn patients and hemorrhages when whole blood is unavailable. |
| **Prednisone** [predniso-lone] | Glucocorti-coid | Used for its immunosuppressant effects and for relief of inflammations; used in arthritis, polymyositis and other systemic diseases. |
| **Pro-Banthine** [propanthe-line bromide] | Anticholin-ergic agent | Used to treat peptic ulcers, GI con-ditions causing spasms and inflam-mation, urethral and bladder spasms, excessive perspiration and enuresis. |
| **Procardia** [nifedipine] | Antianginal agent | Used for management of vasospastic angina and chronic stable angina. |
| **Pronestyl** [procaina-mide hydro-chloride] | Depresses excitability of cardiac muscle | Used in treatment of PVCs, ventricular tachycardia, atrial fibrillation and premature atrial tachycardia (PAT). |
| **Prostigmin** [neostigmine methylsulfate] | Cholinergic-acetyl-cholinest-erase | Used for myasthenia gravis diagnosis and management, amenorrhea, urinary retention, open-angle glaucoma and emergency treatment of angle-closure glaucoma. |
| **Prostin** [dinoprost tromethamin] | Abortifacient | Used for late second trimester abortion. |
| **Quaalude** [methaqua-lone] | Sedative, hypnotic | Used for simple insomnia; induces sleep in patients sensitive to barbitu-rates. |
| **Quinidine, Quinaglute** [quinidine gluconate] | Antiar-rhythmic | Used for management of cardiac arrhythmias. Therapeutic level: 2-5 mcg/ml. Toxic level: > 6 mcg/ml. |
| **Retrovir** (Zidovudine) | Antiretroviral drug | Indicated in symptomatic HIV infection. |

| Drug | Drug Action | Indications |
|------|-------------|-------------|
| **Ritalin** [methyl-phenidate hydrochlo ride] | Central nervous system (CNS) stimulant | Used to overcome depression and hyperkinetic activity in children. |
| **Robaxin** [metho-carbamol] | Muscle relaxant | Used for muscle spasms, bursitis, torti-collis, trauma cases or post-orthopaedic surgery cases. |
| **Robinul** [glycopyrro-late] | Anticholin-ergic, antis-pasmodic | Used in peptic ulcer disease therapy. |
| **Scopolamine** [methscopol-amine bromide] | Anticholin-ergic | Used to treat peptic ulcers, hyper-hidrosis, excessive salivation and selected hypermotile GI conditions. |
| **Seconal** [secobarbital] | Mild seda-tive, hypnotic | Used for minor surgeries, acute convul-sive disorders, and obstetric and dentistry procedures. |
| **Septra DS** [sulfametho-xazole tri-methoprim] | Antibacterial | Used for treatment of urinary tract infections, acute otitis media, acute exacerbations of chronic bronchitis and shigellosis. |
| **Serax** [oxazepam] | Antianxiety | Used for anxiety, tension and alcohol withdrawal. |
| **Sinemet** [carbidopa, levodopa] | Antiparkinso-nian | Used to treat Parkinson's disease. |
| **Slo-Fedrin** [ephedrine sulfate] | Adrenergic agent | Used to treat asthmatic and angion-eurotic conditions, carotid sinus syncope and postural hypotension and to maintain blood pressure during spinal anesthesia. |
| **Solu-Cortef** [hydrocorti-sone sodium succinate] | Antiinflam-matory, adrenocor-tical steroid | Used for treatment of endocrine disor-ders, rheumatic disorders, collagen disease, hematologic disorders. |

| Drug | Drug Action | Indications |
|---|---|---|
| **Solu-Medrol** [methylpred-nisolone sodium succi-nate] | Adrenocor-tico-steroid | Used as antiinflammatory and anti-aller-genic for shock and ulcerative colitis. |
| **Soma** [carisoprodol] | Muscle relaxant | Used for bursitis, lower back disorders, spondylitis, sprains, muscle strains and cerebral palsy. |
| **Sparine** [promazine hydrochlo-ride] | Antipsychotic | Used for DTs, alcoholic hallucinations and drug withdrawal symptoms. |
| **Stadol** [butorphanol tartrate] | Narcotic anal-gesic | Used for moderate to severe post-surgical pain. |
| **Stelazine** [trifluopera-zine] | Antipsy-chotic, anti-emetic | Used to treat schizophrenia; suitable for patients undergoing chemical with-drawal. |
| **Sublimaze** [fentanyl citrate] | Narcotic anal-gesic | Used as analgesic for severe pain, as pre- and postoperative medication; often used for minor surgery for outpa-tients. |
| **Surfak** [dioctyl sodium sulfo-succinate] | Cathartic, emollient | Used to lessen strain of defecation in persons with hernia, cardiovascular compromise or megacolon, or in bedridden cases. |
| **Symmetrel** [amantadine hydrochlo-ride] | Antiparkinso-nian, antiviral | Used in treatment of Parkinson's disease, influenza A virus and respira-tory tract illness. |
| **Synthroid** [levothy-roxine sodium] | Thyroid prep-aration | Used for treatment of hypothyroidism. |

| Drug | Drug Action | Indications |
|------|-------------|-------------|
| **Tagamet** [cimetidine] | Histamine antagonist | Used for treatment of active duodenal ulcer, short-term treatment of active, benign gastric ulcer and treatment of pathological hypersecretory conditions. |
| **Talwin** [pentazocine lactate] | Narcotic analgesic | Used as preoperative sedative and moderate to severe pain reliever. |
| **Tegretol** [carbamazepine] | Anticonvulsant | Used for epilepsy, especially with complex symptomatology. |
| **Tensilon** [edrophonium hydrochloride] | Cholinergic | Used as an adjunct in the evaluation of treatment requirements in myasthenia gravis. |
| **Tessalon** [benzonatate] | Antitussive | Used for respiratory conditions such as pneumonia and bronchitis, and for chronic conditions such as emphysema, tuberculosis, pulmonary tumors and bronchial asthma. |
| **Theo-Dur, Theolair** [theophylline] | Bronchodilator, pulmonary vasodilator, smooth muscle relaxant | Used for treatment of bronchial obstruction in asthma and chronic obstructive pulmonary disease. Therapeutic level: 10-20 mcg/ml. Toxic level: > 20 mcg/ml. |
| **Thiopental sodium** [Pentothal sodium] | Anesthetic agent | Used for preanesthesia or for general anesthesia only. |
| **Thorazine** [chlorpromazine hydrochloride] | Antipsychotic, antiemetic | Used to treat acute and chronic psychoses and alcohol withdrawal, and to control hiccups, nausea and vomiting. |

| Drug | Drug Action | Indications |
|---|---|---|
| **Thrombolysin** [fibrinolysin, human] | Throm-bolytic agent (anticoagu-lant) | Used as modified blood component to dissolve thrombi. |
| **Thytropar** [thyrotropin] | Thyroid prep-aration | Used as diagnostic agent to evaluate thyroid dysfunction. |
| **Tigan** [trimetho-benzamide hydrochlo-ride] | Antiemetic | Used for emesis during surgery, radia-tion-induced nausea and nausea during pregnancy. |
| **Tolectin** [tolmetin sodium] | Antiinflam-matory | Used for rheumatoid arthritis or osteoarthritis. |
| **Tolinase** [tolazamide] | Oral antidia-betic | Used for oral diabetic therapy. |
| **Torecan** [thiethyl-pera-zinemaleate] | Antiemetic | Used to control nausea and vomiting. |
| **Tranxene** [clorazepate dipotassium] | CNS depres-sant | Used for management of anxiety disor-ders, symptomatic relief of acute alcohol withdrawal. |
| **Trinsicon** [ferrous fuma-rate] | Antianemic preparation | Used for treatment of anemias. |
| **Tubocurarine** [tubocurarine chloride] | Natural curare alka-loid | Used for muscle relaxation during abdominal surgery, setting of fractures and dislocations, electroshock therapy and treatment of myasthenia gravis and spasticity caused by injury to CNS. |
| **Urispas** (flavoxate Hcl) | Urinary tract spasmolytic | Used for relief of dysuria, urgency, nocturia, spurapubic pain, frequency and incontinence associated with cystitis, prostatitis, urethritis and ureth-rocystitis/urethrotrigonitis. |

| Drug | Drug Action | Indications |
|------|-------------|-------------|
| **Valium** [diazepam] | Antianxiety, muscle relaxant, anti-convulsant | Used for anxiety, tension, withdrawal from alcohol, muscle spasms and anti-convulsant therapy. |
| **Varidase** [streptoki-nase-streptodor-nase] | Fibrinolytic enzyme | Used for types of pulmonary embolism, deep vein thrombosis, arterial throm-bosis, embolism and coronary artery thrombosis. |
| **Vasoprine** [isoxsuprine hydrochlo-ride] | Peripheral vasodilator | Used to relax vasculature of uterus and to promote cerebrovascular and periph-eral circulation. |
| **Vistaril** [hydroxyzine pamoate] | Antianxiety agent, anti-emetic | Used for treating nausea and vomiting, for reducing narcotic requirement in surgery and as tranquilizer for tension, anxiety or agitation states. |
| **Yutopar** (ritodrine hydrochlo-ride) | Inhibition of contractility of uterine smooth muscles | Used in management of labor in preterm patients. |
| **Zoviraz** (Acyclovir) | Antiviral | Used in treatment of genital herpes and herpes zoster infections. |

# Chapter 5: Most Commonly Missed CC Conditions

| Condition | Documentation |
|---|---|
| **Abscess** | *Signs and Symptoms:* Skin or wound infection. May occur more often in people with poor circulation or diabetes mellitus. Usually begins at site of injury to skin and quickly intensifies. Affected area may be red, hot and swollen.<br><br>*Drug Therapy*— Antibiotics.<br><br>*Laboratory*— Cultures, grain stains and antibiotic sensitivity tests. Blood cultures may be positive.<br><br>*Procedures*— May include punch biopsy or surgical debridement. |
| **Abscess of Bartholin's gland** | *Signs and Symptoms:* Localized pain in region of duct; discomfort when sitting or walking. Organisms causing the infection include Neisseria gonorrhea, E. coli, Streptococcus and Trichomonas vaginalis.<br><br>*Drug Therapy*— Antibiotic therapy.<br><br>*Laboratory*— Smears/cultures: positive for organism causing infection. Blood: possible increase in WBCs.<br><br>*Procedures*— Marsupialization of Bartholin's gland cyst. |
| **Acidosis, respiratory** | *Signs and Symptoms:* Retention of $CO_2$ and increasing $pCO_2$. Hypoventilation, dyspnea, drowsiness, weakness, malaise and nausea.<br><br>*Laboratory*— Arterial blood gases: decreased $CO_2$ (less than 22). Decreased $HCO_2$ (less than 24). Decreased pH (less than 7.35). Increased $pCO_2$ (more than 45). Decreased $pCO_2$ (less than 35). Blood: increased BUN (over 22). Increased potassium (greater than 5.0). Decreased potassium (less than 3.5). Increased chloride (greater than 105). |

| Condition | Documentation |
|---|---|
| **Agranulocytosis** | *Signs and Symptoms:* Bacterial infection and oral ulcerations. Onset is usually acute with fever and chills.<br><br>*Drug Therapy*— Treatment of acute infection with appropriate antibiotics.<br><br>*Laboratory*— Blood: WBC markedly decreased, 95% lymphocytes; RBC and platelets are normal; decreased granulocyte concentration of specific type (i.e., neutropenia, basopenia, eosinopenia). Culture: confirmation of infection.<br><br>*Nurse's Notes*— Protective isolation, frequent monitoring of vital signs. |
| **Alcoholism, acute, continuous** | *Signs and Symptoms:* Alcoholism with acute intoxication. Characteristic physiologic signs are flushed face, slurred speech, unsteady gait and incoordination.<br><br>*Drug Therapy*— B vitamins, antianxiety medications and Antabuse.<br><br>*Laboratory*— Liver enzymes: CPK, LDH, SGOT, SGPT and serum cholesterol may be increased. Blood ethanol level may be increased.<br><br>*Nurse's Notes*— Seizure precautions during withdrawal and documentation of withdrawal symptomatology.<br><br>*Procedures*— Detoxification, group and/or individual therapy.<br><br>*Radiology*— Liver scan and abdominal series. |

| Condition | Documentation |
|---|---|
| **Alcoholism, acute, episodic** | *Signs and Symptoms:* Sometimes maladaptive behavior, aggressiveness and impaired judgment. Characteristic physiologic signs are flushed face, slurred speech, unsteady gait and incoordination.<br><br>*Drug Therapy*— B vitamins, antianxiety medications and Antabuse.<br><br>*Laboratory*— Liver enzymes: CPK, LDH, SGOT, SGPT and serum cholesterol may be increased. Blood ethanol level may be increased.<br><br>*Nurse's Notes*— Seizure precautions during withdrawal and documentation of withdrawal symptomatology.<br><br>*Procedures*— Detoxification and group and/or individual therapy.<br><br>*Radiology*— Liver scan and abdominal series. |
| **Alcoholism, acute, unspecified** | *Signs and Symptoms:* Maladaptive behavior, aggressiveness, impaired judgment. Characteristic physiologic signs are flushed face, slurred speech, unsteady gait and incoordination.<br><br>*Drug Therapy*— B vitamins, antianxiety medications and Antabuse.<br><br>*Laboratory*— Liver enzymes: CPK, LDH, SGOT, SGPT and serum cholesterol may be increased. Blood ethanol level may be increased.<br><br>*Nurse's Notes*— Seizure precautions during withdrawal and documentation of withdrawal symptomatology.<br><br>*Procedures*— Detoxification and group and/or individual therapy.<br><br>*Radiology*— Liver scan and abdominal series. |

| Condition | Documentation |
|-----------|---------------|
| **Alcoholism, chronic, continuous** | *Signs and Symptoms:* Chronic alcohol dependence. Symptoms and signs include delirium tremens, acute alcoholic hallucinations, alcoholic hepatitis or cirrhosis of the liver.<br><br>*Drug Therapy*— B vitamins, antianxiety medications and Antabuse.<br><br>*Laboratory*— Liver enzymes: CPK, LDH, SGOT, SGPT and serum cholesterol may be increased. Blood ethanol level may be increased.<br><br>*Nurse's Notes*— Seizure precautions during withdrawal and documentation of withdrawal symptomatology.<br><br>*Procedures*— Detoxification and group and/or individual therapy.<br><br>*Radiology*— Liver scan and abdominal series. |
| **Alcoholism, chronic, episodic** | *Signs and Symptoms:* Chronic alcohol dependence. Symptoms and signs include delirium tremens, acute alcoholic hallucinations, alcoholic hepatitis or cirrhosis of the liver.<br><br>*Drug Therapy*— B vitamins, antianxiety medications and Antabuse.<br><br>*Laboratory*— Liver enzymes: CPK, LDH, SGOT, SGPT and serum cholesterol may be increased. Blood ethanol level may be increased.<br><br>*Nurse's Notes*— Seizure precautions during withdrawal and documentation of withdrawal symptomatology.<br><br>*Procedures*— Detoxification and group and/or individual therapy<br><br>*Radiology*— Liver scan and abdominal series. |

| Condition | Documentation |
|---|---|
| **Alcoholism, chronic, unspecified** | *Signs and Symptoms:* Chronic alcohol dependence. Symptoms and signs include delirium tremens, acute alcoholic hepatitis or cirrhosis of the liver. |
| | *Drug Therapy—* B vitamins, antianxiety medications and antabuse. |
| | *Laboratory—* Liver enzymes: CPK, LDH, SGOT, SGPT and serum cholesterol may be increased. Blood ethanol level may be increased. |
| | *Nurse's Notes—* Seizure precautions during withdrawal and documentation of withdrawal symptomatology. |
| | *Procedures—* Detoxification and group and/or individual therapy. |
| | *Radiology—* Liver scan and abdominal series. |
| **Alkalosis** | *Signs and Symptoms:* Metabolic alkalosis may show weakness; respiration slow and shallow; uremia. Respiratory alkalosis may show drowsiness, giddiness or paresthesias of the extremities. May be accompanied by a potassium deficiency. |
| | *Laboratory:* Blood (metabolic alkalosis): increased bicarbonate, decreased potassium and increased pH. Blood (respiratory alkalosis): increased bicarbonate excretion, increased pH and decreased $pCO_2$. |
| **Anemia due to acute blood loss** | *Signs and Symptoms:* Rapid, sudden loss of blood following rupture of a peptic ulcer, trauma, hemophilia or an acute leukemia. |
| | *Laboratory—* Blood: hemoglobin less than 8 and hematocrit less than 28. |
| | *Procedures—* Transfusion(s) of blood and blood components. |

| Condition | Documentation |
|---|---|
| **Anemia due to chronic blood loss** | *Signs and Symptoms:* Fatigue, anorexia, dyspnea and irritability. Manifestation often is offset by underlying disease. Pallor, tenderness of bone, functional heart murmur, tachycardia and dilatation of heart.<br><br>*Drug Therapy*— Oral iron medication may be administered.<br><br>*Laboratory*— Blood: RBC decreased, hemoglobin less than 8 and hematocrit less than 28.<br><br>*Procedures*— Bone marrow may be normal, hyperplastic or hypoplastic. |
| **Aneurysm of aorta with rupture** | *Signs and Symptoms:* Can be immediately fatal. Pain is present (constant or paroxysmal) in lower back, groin and possibly testes. Pain is relieved by elevation of knees. Numbness and weakness of legs with occasional paralysis. Cyanosis, syncope and shortness of breath.<br><br>*Drug Therapy*— Nitroprusside IV and narcotics for pain.<br><br>*Nurse's Notes*— Frequent check of vital signs.<br><br>*Procedures*— Surgical management, whole blood transfusion and invasive monitoring.<br><br>*Radiology*— Chest: calcification of aortic wall. Aortography: clinically diagnostic. May show displacement of kidney or ureter. CT scan for confirmation of location. |

| Condition | Documentation |
|---|---|
| **Angina pectoris** | *Signs and Symptoms:* Discomfort in the chest, described as heaviness, pressure, tightness, or squeezing sensation with radiation most usually to the left arm. Underlying disease of ischemia causes interruption of coronary blood flow, creating a lack of oxygen supply to the myocardium. Attacks may be precipitated by emotion, exertion, cold weather, heavy meals or tachycardia. *Drug Therapy*— May include nitroglycerin, isordil or procardia. *EKG*— Normal at first or during rest. Exercise test may show inducing S-T segment depression. *Radiology*— Coronary angiography: evidence of significant obstruction of major coronary artery, myocardial perfusion scans, echocardiography, thallium stress test. |
| **Anorexia nervosa** | *Signs and Symptoms:* Intense fear of obesity resulting in excessive dieting. High level of activity and alertness, associated endocrinologic and physiologic changes and distortion in body image. *Drug Therapy*— Includes medications for correction of nutritional and metabolic deficiencies and psychotherapeutic drugs. *EKG*— Ventricular arrhythmias due to hypokalemia. *Laboratory*— Blood: may show evidence of anemia (hemoglobin less than 8, hematocrit less than 28). *Nurse's Notes*— Intake and output, daily weights and supplemental feedings. *Procedures*— Psychotherapy. |

| Condition | Documentation |
|---|---|
| **Arrest, cardiac** | *Signs and Symptoms:* Sudden unexpected cessation of cardiac action and absence of heart sounds and/or blood pressure. Cardiopulmonary resuscitation performed. <br><br> *Drug Therapy*—May include isoproterenol, atropine, sodium bicarbonate, epinephrine, and calcium gluconate. <br><br> *EKG*— Changes prior to arrest may show bradycardia, tachycardia or other arrhythmias, fibrillation or asystole. <br><br> *Physician's/Nurse's Notes*— Resuscitative efforts recorded in notes or "code" sheet. <br><br> *Procedures*— May include intubation and artificial ventilation. |
| **Ascites** | *Signs and Symptoms:* Fluid accumulation within the peritoneal cavity. <br><br> *Laboratory*— Blood: possible increase in WBC; albumin/globulin ratio possibly reversed. <br><br> *Nurse's Notes*— Daily weights, intake and output and daily abdominal measurements. <br><br> *Procedures*— Paracentesis and insertion of LeVeen Shunt. |
| **Atelectasis** | *Signs and Symptoms:* Known as lung collapse. Symptomatologies vary with amount of parenchyma involved. Dyspnea, cough and possibly orthopnea. <br><br> *Nurse's Notes*— Deep breathing and coughing. Postural drainage (often done by physical therapist). <br><br> *Procedures*— Bronchoscopy, spirometry and nebulizer treatments. <br><br> *Radiology*— Chest x-ray: clinically diagnostic. |

| Condition | Documentation |
|---|---|
| **Bacteremia** | *Signs and Symptoms:* Bacteria in the blood. Elevated temperature and chills and joint pains.<br><br>*Drug Therapy*— Antibiotics depending on organism sensitivity.<br><br>*Laboratory*— Blood culture: positive.<br><br>*Procedures*— IV hydration. |
| **Boils** | *Signs and Symptoms:* Skin infection most commonly found in hairy areas of the body that are subject to heavy perspiration or irritation. Also known as furuncles. Symptoms include localized pain and redness.<br><br>*Drug Therapy*— Topical antibiotics.<br><br>*Laboratory*— Culture: positive for staphylococcus or streptococcus organisms.<br><br>*Nurse's Notes*— Warm compresses.<br><br>*Procedures*— Topical application of moist heat. |
| **Bron-chiectasis** | *Signs and Symptoms:* Irreversible dilation of bronchi, usually resulting from chronic infection. May be congenital or acquired. Production of foul-smelling sputum in large amounts.<br><br>*Drug Therapy*— May include antibiotics for infection and bronchodilators.<br><br>*Laboratory*— Sputum culture: to rule out bacteria or fungi (Aspergillus).<br><br>*Nurse's Notes*— Documentation of postural drainage.<br><br>*Procedures*— Bronchoscopy to determine location and extent of disease and pulmonary function studies.<br><br>*Radiology*— Chest x-ray: rule out tuberculosis and determine fluid level. |

| Condition | Documentation |
|---|---|
| **Bronchitis, chronic** | *Signs and Symptoms:* Persistent cough with usually mucoid tenacious sputum or purulent during infection. Progressive breathlessness or wheezing. Physical examination may document hyperinflation with decreased breath sounds and rhonchi that can be cleared with coughing.<br><br>*Drug Therapy—* May include bronchodilators or antibacterial agents during acute infections and diuretics for edema.<br><br>*EKG—* May show cor pulmonale.<br><br>*Laboratory—* Decreased $pO_2$, increased or normal $pCO_2$.<br><br>*Nurse's Notes—* Postural drainage.<br><br>*Procedures—* $O_2$ therapy and nebulizer treatments.<br><br>*Radiology—* Chest x-ray: hyperinflation with increased bronchovascular markings in acute exacerbations. |
| **Bronchitis, obstructive, chronic** | *Signs and Symptoms:* Bronchitis combined with airway obstruction or emphysema. Advanced disease may be associated with cyanosis with carbon dioxide retention progressing into cor pulmonale.<br><br>*Drug Therapy—* May include both bronchodilators or antibacterial agents and diuretics for edema.<br><br>*Laboratory—* Throat culture: may be positive for organism causing infection.<br><br>*Nurse's Notes—* Postural drainage.<br><br>*Procedures—* $O_2$ therapy and nebulizer treatments.<br><br>*Radiology—* Chest x-ray: clinically diagnostic for obstructive, chronic bronchitis. |

| **Condition** | **Documentation** |
|---|---|
| **Cachexia** | *Signs and Symptoms:* Malnutrition and general ill health marked by emaciation and weakness; usually found in patients with cancer and anorexia nervosa.<br><br>*Drug Therapy*— Vitamin supplements.<br><br>*Laboratory*— Blood chemistry may show nutritional and vitamin deficiencies.<br><br>*Nurse's Notes*— Daily weights, intake and output and supplemental feedings.<br><br>*Procedures*— Total parenteral nutrition (TPN). |
| **Cardiomyop-athy** | *Signs and Symptoms:* Usually demonstrated in elderly patients with loss of consciousness, palpitations and/or dyspnea. Palpitations may be evident by bouncing or rapid pulse and skipped heartbeats.<br><br>*Drug Therapy*— May include digoxin, pronestyl, diuretics and vasodilators.<br><br>*EKG*— May show atrial enlargement, sinus tachycardia, premature ventricular contractions, atrial fibrillation or ventricular hypertrophy.<br><br>*Nurse's Notes*— Intake and output, daily weights, frequent vital signs, documentation of complete bed rest and oxygen therapy.<br><br>*Procedures*— Cardiac catheterization, echocardiogram and possible heart transplant.<br><br>*Radiology*— Chest x-ray may show cardiac hypertrophy and pleural effusion. |
| **Cellulitis** | *Signs and Symptoms:* Skin or wound infection. May occur more often in people with poor circulation or diabetes mellitus. Usually begins at site of injury to skin and quickly intensifies. Affected area may be red, hot and swollen.<br><br>*Drug Therapy*— Antibiotics.<br><br>*Laboratory*— Cultures, grain stains and antibiotic sensitivity tests. Blood cultures may be positive.<br><br>*Procedures*— May include punch biopsy or surgical debridement. |

| Condition | Documentation |
|---|---|
| **Cholangitis** | *Signs and Symptoms:* Pain and discomfort in the right upper quadrant of the abdomen, gradually prolonged. Anorexia, nausea with possible vomiting, chills, pruritus and moderate fever (100.4° to 102.2°F, 38° to 39°C).<br><br>*Laboratory—* Blood: increased WBCs and increased eosinophils.<br><br>*Procedures—* Possible liver biopsy for bile stasis or periportal fibrosis. IV fluids.<br><br>*Radiology—* X-ray: operative cholangiography may show marked narrowing of the choledochal lumen and the extent of involvement of the ducts and radicles.<br><br>*Surgery—* To remove gallbladder and stones |
| **Convulsions** | *Signs and Symptoms:* Sudden, violent, involuntary contraction of a group of muscles that may be episodic or paroxysmal, as in a seizure disorder or following a head trauma.<br><br>*Drug Therapy—* May include dilantin, tegretol, phenobarbital or other anticonvulsant drugs.<br><br>*EEG—* Abnormal; may indicate seizure disorder. |

| Condition | Documentation |
|---|---|
| **Cor pulmonale, acute** | *Signs and Symptoms:* Progressive dyspnea, substernal discomfort or pain, persistent cough, wheezing, fatigue and edema. Documentation of infection. Most commonly results from chronic obstructive pulmonary disease (COPD).<br><br>*Drug Therapy*— May include bronchodilators (e.g., alupent, brethine, aminophylline, bronkosol, epinephrine or theophylline and diuretics, vasodilators, digoxin, antibiotics).<br><br>*EKG*— Cardiac arrhythmias such as premature atrial and ventricular contractions.<br><br>*Laboratory*— Arterial blood gas: may show poor air exchange ($pO_2$ 75-100). Hypoxemia indicated by low $O_2$ saturation ($O_2$ less than 80). Hematocrit often more than 50%.<br><br>*Nurse's Notes*—Intake and output, daily weights, fluid restriction and low-salt diet.<br><br>*Procedures*— Echocardiography or cardiac angiography demonstrating right ventricular hypertrophy.<br><br>*Respiratory Therapy*— May include IPPB treatment, use of $O_2$ (in low concentrations for patients with COPD) and/or use of bronchodilators. Pulmonary function studies. |
| **Cystitis, acute** | *Signs and Symptoms:* An inflammation of the urinary bladder and ureter characterized by urgency, pain, hematuria and frequency of urination caused by calculus, bacterial infections or tumor.<br><br>*Drug Therapy*— May include septra or bactrim and pyridium.<br><br>*Laboratory*— Urinalysis: evidence of WBCs and RBCs in urine. Urine culture: positive. E. coli is the most common organism causing cystitis. |

| Condition | Documentation |
|---|---|
| **Cystitis, chronic** | *Signs and Symptoms:* Prolonged urinary tract infections with long-standing complications of urethral stricture, leukoplakia or urinary retention.<br><br>*Drug Therapy—* May include septra and bactrim.<br><br>*Laboratory—* Urine cultures: may be positive for organism causing infection. Most common is E. coli. Urinalysis: evidence of WBC and RBC. |
| **Dehydration** | *Signs and Symptoms:* Excessive loss of water from the body tissue with a disturbance of the electrolytes, such as sodium, chloride and potassium. Also called volume depletion syndrome.<br><br>*Laboratory—* Blood chemistry may show electrolyte disturbance (i.e., low potassium (less than 3.5)).<br><br>*Nurse's Notes—* Monitoring intake and output. |
| **Disease, Addison's** | *Signs and Symptoms:* Features of crisis include anorexia, headache, weakness, dizziness, nausea, vomiting, apprehension, diarrhea, abdominal pain and syncope. Chronic Addison's disease may show symptoms resembling hypoglycemia (i.e., hunger, sweating, irritability, nervousness and depression).<br><br>*Drug Therapy—* Glucocorticoid and mineralocorticoid replacement.<br><br>*Laboratory—* Blood: sodium and glucose decreased. Potassium level increased. Azotemia present. Plasma cortisol levels decreased. 24 hour urine for 17 ketosteroids and 17 hydroxycorticosteroids to establish baseline urine steroids.<br><br>*Nurse's Notes—* Record of intake and output, weight and vital signs. |

| Condition | Documentation |
|---|---|
| **Disease, hypertensive heart and renal, malignant** | *Signs and Symptoms:* History of renal disease, headache, fatigue and irritability. Evidence of renal failure. Elevated blood pressure (systolic greater than 160 and diastolic greater than 100).<br><br>*Drug Therapy*— Vasodilators such as minoxidil.<br><br>*EKG*— Possible tachycardia.<br><br>*Laboratory*— BUN level greater than 20 and creatinine above 2.5.<br><br>*Nurse's Notes*— Frequent monitoring of vital signs, intake and output and low-sodium diet.<br><br>*Procedures*— Possible kidney transplant and dialysis. |
| **Disease, hypertensive heart, benign, with congestive heart failure** | *Signs and Symptoms:* Elevated blood pressure (systolic greater than 160 and diastolic greater than 100); symptoms may include headache, fatigue, irritability, dyspnea and cardiac arrhythmia.<br><br>*Drug Therapy*— May include aldomet, apresoline, diazide, lopressor, hydroDIURIL, aldactazide or diuril.<br><br>*EKG*— Tachycardia, bradycardia or PVCs.<br><br>*Nurse's Notes*— Frequent monitoring of vital signs, intake and output and oxygen therapy.<br><br>*Procedures*— Ophthalmoscopy: retinopathy.<br><br>*Radiology*— Chest x-ray: may indicate cardiac enlargement. |

| Condition | Documentation |
|---|---|
| **Disease, hypertensive heart, malignant, with congestive heart failure** | *Signs and Symptoms:* Atherosclerosis, history of uncontrolled blood pressure and history of oliguria with varying degrees of renal insufficiency. Onset of elevated blood pressure is usually sudden in nature.<br><br>*Drug Therapy*— May include diuril, hydroDIURIL and reserpine.<br><br>*Laboratory*— BUN greater than 20 and creatinine greater than 2.5.<br><br>*Nurse's Notes*— Frequent monitoring of vital signs with evidence of rapidly accelerated high blood pressure (diastolic greater than 100, systolic greater than 140) and sodium-restricted diet.<br><br>*Procedures*— Ophthalmoscopy: retinopathy.<br><br>*Radiology*— Chest x-ray: congestive heart failure. |
| **Disease, hypertensive heart, unspecified, with congestive heart failure** | *Signs and Symptoms:* Atherosclerosis, obesity, ischemic heart disease, headaches, features of myocardial infarction and paroxysmal nocturnal dyspnea.<br><br>*Drug Therapy*— May include aldactazide, aldomet, inderal, pronestyl, hydroDIURIL or lasix.<br><br>*Nurse's Notes*— Frequent monitoring of vital signs with evidence of high blood pressure (diastolic greater than 100, systolic greater than 140).<br><br>*Procedures*— Ophthalmoscopy: retinopathy and papilledema.<br><br>*Radiology*— Chest x-ray: congestive heart failure and cardiac enlargement. |

| Condition | Documentation |
|---|---|
| **Disease, pelvic inflamma- tory, acute (PID)** | *Signs and Symptoms:*  Also known as "PID." Neisseria gonorrhoeae is the most common causative organism. Sexually transmitted in the cervix. Symptoms include profuse vaginal discharge, lower abdominal pain and low-grade fever.<br><br>*Drug Therapy—*  May include pain medications and agents selected specifically for treatment of the organism causing PID. For PID caused by gonorrhea, penicillin G procaine IM is the drug of choice.<br><br>*Laboratory—*  Vaginal gram stain and cultures: positive.<br><br>*Procedures—*  Culdocentesis for fluid or pus for culture and sensitivity. Ultrasonography, which demonstrates an adnexal or uterine mass. |
| **Disease, pulmonary, obstructive, chronic (COPD)** | *Signs and Symptoms:*  Irreversible and progressive condition characterized by diminished inspiratory and expiratory capacity of the lungs.<br><br>*Drug Therapy—*  May include bronchodilators or antibiotics in acute infections.<br><br>*Laboratory—*  Arterial blood gases: $pO_2$ is usually lower than normal and $pCO_2$ is usually higher than normal.<br><br>*Radiology—*  Chest x-ray:  emphysema predominating and increased lung size. |
| **Effusion, pleural** | *Signs and Symptoms:*  Collection of fluid in the pleura. Dry cough, signs of congestion, tachycardia, dyspnea and possible pleuritic pain.<br><br>*Drug Therapy—*  May include a diuretic agent such as Lasix or digoxin.<br><br>*Procedures—*  Thoracentesis.<br><br>*Radiology—*  Chest x-ray:  usually diagnostic of this condition. |

| Condition | Documentation |
|---|---|
| **Emphysema** | *Signs and Symptoms:* Manifestations modified by influences of associated pulmonary disease, condition, exertional dyspnea, cough, wheezing and weakness.<br><br>*Drug Therapy*— May include bronchodilators (e.g., alupent, brethine, aminophylline).<br><br>*Laboratory*— Arterial blood gases: evidence of $CO_2$ retention.<br><br>*Radiology*— Chest x-ray: radiolucency of lung during full expiration. Possible accentuation of hilar marking.<br><br>*Respiratory Therapy*— Pulmonary function: vital capacity reduced. Low-flow oxygen therapy. |
| **Endometritis (acute)** | *Signs and Symptoms:* Features of salpingitis and vaginal discharge.<br><br>*Drug Therapy*— May include appropriate antibiotics and possibly vaginal creams.<br><br>*Laboratory*— Increased WBC. Vaginal smear: positive. Culture of vaginal discharge: positive. |

| Condition | Documentation |
|---|---|
| **Failure, heart, congestive (CHF)** | *Signs and Symptoms:* Dyspnea is present with orthopnea and paroxysmal nocturnal dyspnea present in more advanced failure. Other symptoms include peripheral edema, irritability and weakness. Cyanosis is present on occasion. Heart rate is irregular. Moist rales are present in bases of lungs with productive cough. Confusion is usually present. |
| | *Drug Therapy*— May include digoxin, diuretics and vasodilators. |
| | *EKG*— Tachycardia and atrial enlargement. |
| | *Laboratory*— Possible increase in plasma volume above 5% of body weight. |
| | *Nurse's Notes*— Frequent monitoring of vital signs, intake and output, antiembolism hose, low-sodium diet, oxygen therapy, daily weights, fluid restriction and rotating tourniquets. |
| | *Procedures*— Echocardiography, cardiac blood pool imaging, pulmonary artery monitoring and cardiac catheterization. |
| | *Radiology*— Chest x-ray: may show cardiac hypertrophy, pleural effusion or pulmonary venous congestion. |
| **Fibrillation, atrial** | *Signs and Symptoms:* Occurs as a result of other conditions, such as congestive heart failure and sepsis, or after bypass or valve replacement surgery. Symptoms include palpitations, dyspnea, dizziness, fainting and apprehension. |
| | *Drug Therapy*— May include digoxin, diuretics and quinidine. |
| | *EKG*— Atrial rate over 400/minute with a variable ventricular rate. Absence of P waves. |
| | *Procedures*— Cardioversion and echocardiography. |

| Condition | Documentation |
|---|---|
| **Failure, renal** | *Signs and Symptoms:* Lethargy, fatigue, anorexia, nausea, dyspnea, weakness, thirst, oliguria, bradycardia or tachycardia and hematuria.<br><br>*EKG*— Arrhythmias of all types due to electrolyte imbalance.<br><br>*Laboratory*— Urinalysis: low specific gravity, high specific gravity if due to prerenal or postrenal factors, RBC, protein; traces of glucose, casts, epithelial cells. Blood: increase in WBCs during infection; increase of BUN and creatinine.<br><br>*Nurse's Notes*— Daily weights and intake and output.<br><br>*Procedures*— Dialysis. |
| **Failure, respiratory** | *Signs and Symptoms:* Inability of the pulmonary and cardiac systems to maintain an adequate exchange of carbon dioxide and oxygen in the lungs. Acute respiratory failure (ARF) is a life- threatening emergency. Symptoms include increase in sputum production, cough and shortness of breath.<br><br>*Laboratory*— Arterial blood gases: increased $pCO_2$ (greater than 50) and decreased $pO_2$ (less than 50).<br><br>*Procedures*— $O_2$ therapy and artificial ventilation.<br><br>*Radiology*— Chest x-ray: may show congestion caused by an infectious process or an obstructive process such as emphysema or chronic obstructive pulmonary disease. |

| Condition | Documentation |
|---|---|
| **Fibrillation, ventricular** | *Signs and Symptoms:* A life-threatening cardiac emergency. Absence of effective cardiac action resulting in loss of pulse, respirations and blood pressure. Seizures and death can occur. <br><br> *Drug Therapy*— Lidocaine, procainamide and bretylium tosylate. <br><br> *EKG*— Bizarre (QRS) complexes; ventricular rhythm chaotic and rapid. <br><br> *Nurse's Notes*— CPR and oxygen therapy. <br><br> *Procedures*— Cardiopulmonary resuscitation and defibrillation. drawal and documentation of withdrawal symptomatology. <br><br> *Procedures*— Detoxification and group and/or individual therapy. <br><br> *Radiology*— Liver scan and abdominal series. |
| **Fistula of bladder** | *Signs and Symptoms:* Urinary incontinence, dysuria and vaginal irritation. <br><br> *Drug Therapy*— May include antibiotic therapy. <br><br> *Procedures*— Cystoscopy. Surgery to repair fistula. |
| **Flutter, atrial** | *Signs and Symptoms:* Palpitation, weakness, dizziness, syncope anxiety and feeling of impending death. <br><br> *Drug Therapy*— May include digoxin, quinidine, propranolol. <br><br> *EKG*— P waves in regular rhythm (250-350 per minute) and PR interval prolonged, varying with degree of AV block. <br><br> *Nurse's Notes*— Documentation of rapid, regular atrial rate between 220 and 360 per minute. <br><br> *Procedures*— Cardioversion, atrial pacemaker and vagal stimulation. |

| Condition | Documentation |
|---|---|
| **Fracture, pathological** | *Signs and Symptoms:* Fracture resulting in weakened bone tissue. Pain, swelling, discoloration and tenderness at fracture site.<br><br>*Procedures—* Surgery to reduce and immobilize fracture. Traction and wound care may be necessary.<br><br>*Radiology—* Skeletal x-ray: diagnostic of pathological fracture. CAT scan and MRI. |
| **Hematemesis** | *Signs and Symptoms:* Vomiting of blood or "coffee ground material."<br><br>*Drug Therapy—* May include vasopressin.<br><br>*Laboratory—* Stool may show blood in specimen. May show decreased hemoglobin and hematocrit.<br><br>*Nurse's Notes—* Frequent monitoring of vital signs and intake and output.<br><br>*Procedures—* IV therapy for volume replacement and endoscopy.<br><br>*Radiology—* X rays may include uppergastrointestinal to determine source of hemorrhage, arteriography and nuclear scans. |
| **Hematuria** | *Signs and Symptoms:* Blood in the urine.<br><br>*Drug Therapy—* May include agents for treatment of underlying cause (e.g., urinary tract infection) (septra or bactrim).<br><br>*Laboratory—* Urinalysis: red blood cells in urine specimen, indicating hemorrhage or infectious process. Blood: elevated erythrocyte sedimentation rate (ESR). |

| Condition | Documentation |
|---|---|
| **Hemorrhage, gastrointestinal** | *Signs and Symptoms:* May be evident by vomiting of blood or signs of blood in stool (black and tarry).<br><br>*Laboratory—* Stool may show blood in specimen. May show decreased hemoglobin and hematrocrit.<br><br>*Nurse's Notes—* Frequent monitoring of vital signs and intake and output.<br><br>*Procedures—* Endoscopy and colonoscopy.<br><br>*Radiology—* X-rays may include upper and lower gastrointestinal tract studies to determine source of bleeding. |
| **Hydrocele, infected** | *Signs and Symptoms:* Inflammation, infection of the spermatic cord or testis.<br><br>*Laboratory—* Culture: fluid fibrinous, purulent or hemorrhagic, depending on underlying disease. |
| **Hyponatremia** | *Signs and Symptoms:* Less than normal amount of sodium in the blood, caused by inadequate excretion of water or by excessive water in the circulating bloodstream due to vomiting, diarrhea, cirrhosis or drugs such as diuretics. Symptoms include muscle cramps, lethargy, nausea and seizures.<br><br>*Laboratory—* Blood chemistry: low sodium.<br><br>*Nurse's Notes—* Intake and output. |
| **Ileus, paralystic (adynamic)** | *Signs and Symptoms:* Vomiting, cramps, pain, abdominal distention.<br><br>*Procedures—* Nasogastric (NG) tube to remove intestinal contents. Miller-Abbott tube to decompress the intestine.<br><br>*Nurse's Notes—* Monitoring of pulse, BP and urine flow.<br><br>*Radiology—* Plain abdominal x-ray will show gas in the small intestine. |

| Condition | Documentation |
|---|---|
| **Infarction, myocardial, acute** | *Signs and Symptoms:* Deep severe substernal pain with radiation to back, jaw or left arm. Pain may be mild or even unrecognized in some patients. Unresponsive to nitroglycerin. May be preceded by angina pectoris. Signs of left heart failure may be predominant. Arrhythmias and apprehension may often accompany the acute myocardial infarction. |
| | *Drug Therapy—* May include use of morphine IM or intravenous to relieve pain. Antiarrhythmic medication may also be administered, such as lidocaine. |
| | *EKG—* Evidence of acute ischemia and infarction pattern. |
| | *Laboratory—* Cardiac enzymes: increased CPK, SGOT, LDH, CK-MB and/or LD-1 fractions. |
| | *Nurse's Notes—* Intake and output and cardiopulmonary resuscitation in the event of cardiac arrest. |
| | *Procedures—* Coronary angiography and $O_2$ therapy. |
| **Infection of urinary tract** | *Signs and Symptoms:* Dysuria or pain on urination, frequency of urination and sometimes retention of urine. Fever, chills, general malaise and hematuria. |
| | *Drug Therapy—* Appropriate antibiotic. |
| | *Laboratory—* Urinalysis: WBC, RBC and bacteria. Urine culture: positive for organism causing infection. |

| Condition | Documentation |
|---|---|
| **Ischemia, coronary, acute and subacute** | *Signs and Symptoms:* Arteriosclerotic heart disease, elevated cholesterol, disease of aortic valve, thoracic pain, anemia, dizziness, syncope and dyspnea.<br><br>*Drug Therapy*— May include nitroglycerin, lidocaine, pronestyl, digoxin, quinidine, and potassium supplement administered intravenously.<br><br>*EKG*— Documentation may indicate subacute ischemia.<br><br>*Laboratory*— Potassium: may show a decrease in level indicating cardiac damage. Enzymes: slightly elevated cholesterol level greater than 250. Anemia (hemoglobin less than 8 and hematocrit less than 28).<br><br>*Nurse's Notes*— May document cardiac monitoring or CCU services.<br><br>*Procedures*— Stress EKG and cardiac catheterization.<br><br>*Radiology*— Echocardiogram, myocardial perfusion studies and gated blood pool imaging. Chest x-ray may show cardiac enlargement and increased hilar markings. |
| **Malnutrition (protein–calorie)** | *Signs and Symptoms:* Weakness, emaciation, loss of subcutaneous fat and multiple vitamin deficiencies. Increased likelihood of infections and other disease processes. Can result in electrolyte imbalances.<br><br>*Drug Therapy*— May include hydration and vitamin supplements. Other supplements may include potassium.<br><br>*Laboratory*— Blood: may be indicative of iron deficiency anemia, low vitamin levels and low protein levels.<br><br>*Nurse's Notes*— Intake and ouput and dietary supplements.<br><br>*Procedures*— TTPN<br><br>*Radiology*— X-ray: decreased mineralization of bone. |

| Condition | Documentation |
|---|---|
| **Melena** | *Signs and Symptoms:* Black, tarry stools with digested blood.<br><br>*Laboratory*— Stool may show blood in specimen. May show decreased hemoglobin and hematocrit.<br><br>*Nurse's Notes*— Frequent monitoring of vital signs and intake and output.<br><br>*Procedures*— Sigmoidoscopy and colonoscopy.<br><br>*Radiology*— X-ray may include upper and/or lower gastrointestinal tract to determine source of hemorrhage and may include barium enema, angiogram and nuclear scans. |
| **Myocarditis, acute** | *Signs and Symptoms:* Inflammation of the myocardium caused by viral, bacterial or fungal infection. Precordial or substernal discomfort with severe dyspnea and later, abdominal discomfort in the right upper quadrant. Rapidly progressive clinical course can be complicated by congestive heart failure.<br><br>*Drug Therapy*— May include antiarrhythmic drugs to control arrhythmias, antibiotics for underlying infection and antiinflammatory drugs.<br><br>*EKG*— Tachycardia, intraventricular or bundle branch abnormalities.<br><br>*Laboratory*— CPK, SGOT and LDH may be elevated. Viral antibody titers, WBCs and erythrocyte sedimentation rates are also elevated.<br><br>*Nurse's Notes*— Oxygen therapy, frequent vital signs and documentation of bed rest.<br><br>*Procedures*— Endomyocardial biopsy and echocardiogram.<br><br>*Radiology*— Chest x-ray: cardiac enlargement. |

| Condition | Documentation |
|---|---|
| **Myositis, infective** | *Signs and Symptoms:* Pain in muscles, possible fever and chills with muscle swelling.<br><br>*Laboratory—* Blood: CBCs, WBCs, ESR and eosinophils elevated.<br><br>*Radiology—* Arteriography may show displacement of arteries and abnormal vascular patterns. |
| **Neuritis or radiculitis, brachial** | *Signs and Symptoms:* Weakness of neck, inside forearm and shoulder. This can sometimes occur after an injection of tetanus or diphtheria antitoxins.<br><br>*Radiology—* X-ray: cervical and shoulder. Possible bone scan. |
| **Obstruction, urinary** | *Signs and Symptoms:* Unable to urinate and feeling of not emptying. Pain, hematuria and changes in urinary output.<br><br>*Drug Therapy—* May include agents such as bactrim or septra and analgesics for pain.<br><br>*Procedures—* Cystoscopy may be performed to diagnose obstruction or as a means to remove the obstruction.<br><br>*Radiology—* X-ray: may be diagnostic of obstruction. Plain abdominal films would be followed by an intravenous pyelogram (IVP). |
| **Orchitis with abscess** | *Signs and Symptoms:* Inflammation and infection of testes. Area may be reddened and tender.<br><br>*Drug Therapy—* Antibiotic therapy and diethylstilbestrol (DES) for mumps or orchitis.<br><br>*Laboratory—* Blood: WBCs may be elevated. Culture: positive.<br><br>*Nurse's Notes—* Bed rest and ice pack to scrotum. |

| Condition | Documentation |
|---|---|
| **Pancreatitis (acute)** | *Signs and Symptoms:* Damage to the biliary tract by alcohol, infectious disease, trauma or certain drugs. Jaundice will occur in patients with common bile duct obstruction. Continuous pain in the epigastric area and sometimes referred to the back. Abdomen is distended and tender. Fever is present.<br><br>*Drug Therapy*— May include large doses of antibiotics and drugs to control pain.<br><br>*Laboratory*— Blood: WBCs are elevated as well as amylase, leucine aminopeptidase, bilirubin and lipase.<br><br>*Procedures*— Intravenous hydration and nasogastric tube for suction.<br><br>*Radiology*— X-ray: stomach and duodenum are displaced, and calcification of pancreas in evident. CAT scan to identify presence and extent of pancreatitis. |

| Condition | Documentation |
|---|---|
| **Pericarditis, acute, unspecified** | *Signs and Symptoms:* Onset is usually abrupt and often preceded by sharp precordial or substernal pain, radiating to the neck. Precordial pain can be distinguished from ischemic coronary pain because it usually is not aggravated by thoracic motion. Fever, chills and weakness are common.<br><br>*Drug Therapy*— Intravenous antibiotics, corticosteroids and antiinflammatory drugs such as aspirin and Indocin.<br><br>*EKG*— Tachycardia, S-T segment elevation and atrial arrhythmias.<br><br>*Laboratory*— WBC count 15,000-20,000, SGOT increased (above 40 units), and PPD skin test is positive if caused by tuberculosis. Positive gram stain and positive culture.<br><br>*Nurse's Notes*— Documentation of complete bed rest, frequent monitoring of vital signs and oxygen therapy.<br><br>*Procedures*— Pericardiocentesis: fluid may be hemorrhagic or straw-colored. Echocardiogram if pericardial effusion is present.<br><br>*Radiology*— Chest x-ray: usually serial for the purpose of ruling out cause of pleuritic chest pain. May show slight cardiac hypertrophy. |
| **Peritonitis** | *Signs and Symptoms:* Inflammation of the peritoneum caused by acute irritating substances or bacteria entering the abdominal cavity by perforation of an organ in the gastrointestinal tract, the reproductive tract or a penetrating wound. Abdominal pain with nausea and vomiting, and chills.<br><br>*Drug Therapy*—IV antibiotics such as doxycycline, cefoxitin, clindamycin and gentamicin.<br><br>Laboratory—Blood: elevated WBCs. Positive gram strain and positive culture.<br><br>*Nurse's Notes*—Documentation of abdominal distention, ascites and possibly elevated temperature.<br><br>Radiology—Abdominal x-ray: ileus. |

| Condition | Documentation |
|---|---|
| **Phlebitis and thrombophlebitis of femoral vein** | *Signs and Symptoms:* Inflammation of a vein generally followed by a clot. Affected area may be hot and tender to touch. Other symptoms include swelling of the extremity, pain and cyanosis. <br><br> *Drug Therapy*— May include heparin given intravenously or subcutaneously followed by a course of oral anticoagulants. <br><br> *Laboratory*— Increase in platelet and leucocyte count. Frequent APTT monitoring. <br><br> *Radiology*— X-ray: may be diagnostic of the affected area. Arteriography: may be diagnostic of location of thrombus. |
| **Phlebitis and thrombophlebitis of superficial vessels, lower extremities** | *Signs and Symptoms:* Inflammation of vein generally followed by a clot. May be hot and tender to touch. <br><br> *Drug Therapy*— May include administration of anticoagulant agent such as heparin. <br><br> *Radiology*— X-ray: may be diagnostic of the affected area. Arteriography: may be diagnostic of the location of the clot. |
| **Pneumonia** | *Signs and Symptoms:* Lung infection may be due to a number of organisms that may cause the infection. Symptoms include cough, fever, chills and sometimes general aching. <br><br> *Drug Therapy*— Appropriate antibiotic therapy is usually given according to organism. <br><br> *Laboratory*— Blood: elevated WBCs. Culture (sputum) is positive for: Haemophilus influenzae, klebsiella, pseudomonas, staphylococcus, streptococcus or other specified bacteria. <br><br> *Nurse's Notes*— Oxygen therapy and analgesics for chest pain. <br><br> *Procedures*— May include bronchoscopy. <br><br> *Radiology*— Chest x-ray may show infiltrates. |

| Condition | Documentation |
|---|---|
| **Pneu-mothorax** | *Signs and Symptoms:* Collapse of the lung caused by the collection of air in the pleural space. Usually sudden in onset; pain in chest on involved side, radiating to neck. Cough and rapid onset of severe dyspnea. Cyanosis and asymmetrical chest wall movement also present.<br><br>*Procedures—* Oxygen therapy.<br><br>*Radiology—* X-ray: outline of collapsed lung. Mediastinal shift to opposite side.<br><br>*Respiratory Therapy—* Pulmonary function: vital capacity decreased.<br><br>*Surgery—* Chest tube placement. |
| **Prostatitis, acute** | *Signs and Symptoms:* Inflammation of the prostate gland caused by infection. Dysuria, frequency, urgency, burning and painful urination.<br><br>*Drug Therapy—* May include appropriate antibiotic.<br><br>*Laboratory—* Urinalysis: evidence of WBC, RBC and bacteria. Urine culture may identify organism causing infection.<br><br>*Nurse's Notes—* Force fluids and sitz baths.<br><br>*Procedures—* Possible suprapubic cystostomy. |
| **Retention, urinary** | *Signs and Symptoms:* Acquired obstruction or a congenital defect. Patient is unable to urinate or completely empty bladder. May also be due to a neurological disorder, such as multiple sclerosis, or trauma, such as a spinal cord injury.<br><br>*Drug Therapy—* May include bactrim or septra.<br><br>*Nurse's Notes—* Documentation of residual urine volume and intake and output. Also bladder training.<br><br>*Procedures—* Cystoscopy may be performed to determine reason for obstruction. Cystometrogram to measure pressure and capacity of bladder.<br><br>*Radiology—* IVP may be performed for diagnostic purposes. |

| Condition | Documentation |
|---|---|
| **Seizure, Petit mal, with intractable epilepsy** | *Signs and Symptoms:* Momentary loss of memory with twitching face and upper extremities. May be characterized by momentary staring into space. Also known as "absence seizure." |
| | *Drug Therapy*— May include dilantin or phenobarbital. |
| | *EEG*— Diagnostic. |
| **Septicemia** | *Signs and Symptoms:* Chills, skin eruptions, fever, nausea, vomiting, diarrhea and prostration. |
| | *Drug Therapy*— Antibiotics. |
| | *Laboratory*— Blood cultures; serial white blood cell counts, between 15,000 and 30,000 with a left shift. Platelet count decreased. BUN and creatinine are increased. |

| Condition | Documentation |
|---|---|
| **Shock, cardiogenic** | *Signs and Symptoms:* A life-threatening emergency requiring intensive stabilizing measures. Most often occurs as the result of a myocardial infarction, end-stage cardiomyopathy or possibly a malfunction of the mitral valve. Rapidly developing mental confusion with weakness, cyanosis, oliguria, tachycardia and gallop rhythm. Systolic pressure drops to 50. Skin is cool and moist.<br><br>*Drug Therapy*—May include morphine to control chest pain, dopamine, norepinephrine and nitroprusside.<br><br>*EKG*— Ventricular fibrillation may be present.<br><br>*Laboratory*— May show serum acidosis. BUN and creatinine are elevated, as are CPK, LDH, SGOT and SGPT. Arterial blood gases demonstrate acidosis and hypoxia.<br><br>*Nurse's Notes*— May indicate a weak rapid pulse, cardiac monitoring and intake and output.<br><br>*Procedures*— Pulmonary artery pressure monitoring (PAP) and pulmonary capillary wedge pressure (PCWP). May also include intraaortic balloon pump (IABP).<br><br>*Radiology*— Chest x-ray may show pulmonary edema. |

| Condition | Documentation |
|---|---|
| **Shock, septic** | *Signs and Symptoms:* May include septic shock due to management of underlying disease. Hypotension and fever may be present except in chronically ill or elderly patients. Onset of abrupt chills, nausea, vomiting and diarrhea. Documentation of extreme exhaustion (prostration). |
| | *Drug Therapy*— Dopamine for renal perfusion, IV antibiotics. |
| | *EKG*— May demonstrate conduction defect and/or ventricular fibrillation. |
| | *Laboratory*— Blood: may show acidosis or elevated BUN and creatinine, leukocytosis or neutropenia. |
| | *Procedures*— Invasive monitoring with a pulmonary artery catheter. |
| | *Radiology*— Chest x-ray: may show pulmonary edema. |
| **Tachycardia, paroxysmal, supraventricular** | *Signs and Symptoms:* Abrupt onset and termination of palpitations. Often asymptomatic although patient may be aware of a rapid heartbeat. Some patients complain of throbbing vessels of the throat, dyspnea, sweating, dizziness, syncope, weakness and polyuria. |
| | *Drug Therapy*— May include propranolol, quinidine or verapamil. |
| | *EKG*— Premature atrial beats, abnormally shaped P waves. Regular rhythm at 150-220 beats per minute. |
| | *Procedures*— May include intracardiac electrophysiologic studies and vagal stimulation. May also see reduced vital capacity and increased cardiac output and circulation time. |
| **Tachycardia, paroxysmal, unspecified** | *Signs and Symptoms:* Fluttering sensation in the chest, weakness, faintness and nausea. |
| | *Drug Therapy*— May include quinidine, procainamide, tambocor, disopyramide. |
| | *EKG*— Uninterrupted series of beats. |

| **Condition** | **Documentation** |
|---|---|
| **Tachycardia, paroxysmal, ventricular** | *Signs and Symptoms:* Associated with ischemic heart disease, especially myocardial infarction. Precordial pain. Sudden onset usually preceded by premature ventricular beats. Pulse rate of 150-210 per minute. *Drug Therapy*— May include antiarrhythmic medication (e.g., lidocaine, pronestyl). *EKG*— Wide QRS complexes. *Nurse's Notes*— Cardiopulmonary resuscitation. *Procedures*— Cardioversion. |
| **Ulcer, decubitus** | *Signs and Symptoms:* Also known as a bedsore or pressure sore. Occurs most frequently in debilitated patients who are bed- or wheelchair-confined. Is a result of loss of circulation to a susceptible body area, such as a bony prominence. *Drug Therapy*— May include topical antibiotic ointments. *Nurse's Notes*— May show special mattresses used for treatment and prevention of spread of ulcer, dressing changes and treatment of decubitus. *Procedures*— Fourth stage ulcers may be debrided. Whirlpool debridements in physical therapy may be required. |
| **Varices, esophageal, bleeding** | *Signs and Symptoms:* Hematemesis can sometimes be an indication of an esophageal bleed. *Drug Therapy*— Peripheral venous or central arterial vasopressin. *Procedures*— Esophagoscopy: diagnostic. Barium swallow: diagnostic. Balloon tamponade. *Surgery*— Endoscopic sclerosis of bleeding varices. |

# Chapter 6: Cardiovascular Complications

| Condition | Documentation |
|---|---|
| **Aneurysm of aorta, dissecting, any part** | *Signs and Symptoms:* Severe pain in anterior part of chest, possibly back, lumbar area and abdomen. Nausea, weakness of legs, unconsciousness and intermittent claudication. Condition is an extreme emergency necessitating emergency surgery and invasive monitoring and intensive stabilizing measures.<br><br>*History & Physical Exam*— Pulsation of lower extremities.<br><br>*Nurse's Notes*— Documentation of increased blood pressure. Oxygen therapy blood transfusion and invasive monitoring.<br><br>*Procedures*— Pulmonary capillary wedge pressure and central venous pressure.<br><br>*Radiology*— CAT scan to confirm size and location, aortography, MRI; widening of aortic shadow. Arteriography: calcification |
| **Aneurysm of coronary vessels** | *Signs and Symptoms:* Distressing cardiac palpitation. Severe dyspnea. Generalized edema.<br><br>*Radiology*— Chest x-ray: cardiac enlargement. Arteriography: calcifications. |

| Condition | Documentation |
|---|---|
| **Aneurysm of heart** | *Signs and Symptoms:* Distressing cardiac palpitation. Severe dyspnea. Generalized edema. Shock can occur after myocardial infarction.<br><br>*Drug Therapy*— May include anitarrhythmics such as procainamide, quinidine or disopyramide.<br><br>*EKG*— Bundle branch abnormality, possible T wave changes; S-T segment elevated.<br><br>*Nurse's Notes*— Frequent monitoring of vital signs and intake and output, and cardiopulmonary resuscitation.<br><br>*Procedures*— Cardioversion.<br><br>*Radiology*— Chest x-ray: enlarged heart with dilation, possibly localized calcification. Ventriculography: reduced cardiac output and hypertrophy of left ventricle. |
| **Arrest, cardiac** | *Signs and Symptoms:* Sudden unexpected cessation of cardiac action, absence of heart sounds and/or blood pressure. Cardiopulmonary resuscitation performed.<br><br>*Drug Therapy*— May include isoproterenol, atropine, sodium bicarbonate, epinephrine and calcium gluconate.<br><br>*EKG*— Bradycardia, tachycardia; S-T segment deviation, fibrillation or asystole.<br><br>*Physician's/Nurse's Notes*— Resuscitative efforts recorded in notes or "code sheet."<br><br>*Procedures*— May include intubation and artificial ventilation. |
| **Block, atrio-ventricular** | *Signs and Symptoms:* Dyspnea, faintness and weakness.<br><br>*Drug Therapy*— Atropine may be given.<br><br>*EKG*— Various patterns producing an irregularly dropped beat can be determined by cardiac auscultation or palpation of the pulse. |

| Condition | Documentation |
|---|---|
| **Block, atrio-ventricular, complete (third-degree block)** | *Signs and Symptoms:* Also called "complete" heart block. Atrioventricular disassociation, complete. Possible angina pectoris. Exertional dyspnea, dizziness, palpitation and possible syncope.<br><br>*Drug Therapy*— Isoproterenol or epinephrine.<br><br>*EKG*— Focus below bifurcation; premature ventricular beats.<br><br>*Procedures*— Insertion of temporary pacemaker followed by a permanent pacemaker. |
| **Block, atrio-ventricular, Mobitz type I, second degree** | *Signs and Symptoms:* Also called "partial" or "incomplete" heart block. Weakness, faintness, palpitation and dyspnea transient when in upright position. Usually transient in nature and requires no treatment.<br><br>*Drug Therapy*— Atropine for bradycardia.<br><br>*EKG*— Often documented as "Wenckebach" pause. Irregular ventricular rhythm, regular atrial rhythm.<br><br>*Procedures*— Temporary pacemaker. |
| **Block, atrio-ventricular, Mobitz type II** | *Signs and Symptoms:* Also called "partial" or "incomplete" heart block. Attack of syncope related to sudden cessation of circulation in upright or recumbent position.<br><br>*Drug Therapy*— Atropine for bradycardia. Discontinue digitalis.<br><br>*EKG*— Block may be documented as 2:1, 3:1, or 4:1. Sudden onset of AV disassociation.<br><br>*Procedures*— Temporary pacemaker and permanent pacemaker if necessary. |
| **Block, bilateral bundle branch** | *Signs and Symptoms:* Symptoms are usually absent.<br><br>*EKG*— QRS duration of 0.12 seconds or more. Diastolic gallop rhythm. |

| Condition | Documentation |
|-----------|---------------|
| **Block, left bundle branch** | *Signs and Symptoms:* Symptoms are usually absent. Usually secondary to coronary artery disease or hypertension. Makes the diagnosis of acute myocardial infarction more difficult.<br><br>*EKG—* QRS duration of 0.12 seconds or more and contour of complex is distorted. Diastolic gallop rhythm. |
| **Block, right bundle branch and left anterior fascicular block** | *Signs and Symptoms:* Symptoms are usually absent.<br><br>*EKG—* Left anterior fascicular block. QRS complex lasting 0.12 seconds or longer. T wave essentially normal in all leads except V1-V3. |
| **Block, right bundle branch and left posterior fascicular block** | *Signs and Symptoms:* Symptoms are usually absent. Occurs less frequently than left anterior fascicular block.<br><br>*EKG—* Left posterior fascicular block. QRS complex lasting 0.12 seconds or longer. T wave essentially normal in all leads except V1-V3. |
| **Block, trifascicular** | *Signs and Symptoms:* Dizziness, syncope, dyspnea and weakness.<br><br>*EKG—* Combined arrhythmias. |
| **Disease, hypertensive heart, benign, with congestive heart failure** | *Signs and Symptoms:* Elevated blood pressure (systolic greater than 160 and diastolic greater than 100). Symptoms may include headache, fatigue, irritability, dyspnea and cardiac arrhythmia.<br><br>*Drug Therapy—* May include aldomet, apresoline, diazide, lopressor, hydroDIURIL, aldactazide or diuril.<br><br>*EKG—* Tachycardia, bradycardia or PVCs.<br><br>*Nurse's Notes—* Frequent monitoring of vital signs and intake and output, and oxygen therapy.<br><br>*Procedures—* Ophthalmoscopy: retinopathy.<br><br>*Radiology—* Chest x-ray: may indicate cardiac enlargement. |

| Condition | Documentation |
|---|---|
| **Disease, hypertensive heart, malignant, with congestive heart failure** | *Signs and Symptoms:* Atherosclerosis, history of uncontrolled blood pressure and history of oliguria with varying degrees of renal insufficiency. Onset of elevated blood pressure is usually sudden in nature.<br><br>*Drug Therapy*— May include diuril, hydroDIURIL, reserpine.<br><br>*Laboratory*— BUN greater than 20, creatinine greater than 2.5.<br><br>*Nurse's Notes*— Frequent monitoring of vital signs, with evidence of rapidly accelerated high blood pressure (diastolic greater than 100, systolic greater than 140), and sodium-restricted diet.<br><br>*Procedures*— Ophthalmoscopy: retinopathy.<br><br>*Radiology*— Chest x-ray: congestive heart failure. |
| **Disease, hypertensive heart, unspecified, with congestive heart failure** | *Signs and Symptoms:* Atherosclerosis, obesity, ischemic heart disease, headaches, features of myocardial infarction and paroxysmal nocturnal dyspnea.<br><br>*Drug Therapy*— May include aldactazide, aldomet, inderal, pronestyl, hydroDIURIL or lasix.<br><br>*Nurse's Notes*— Frequent monitoring of vital signs, with evidence of high blood pressure (diastolic greater than 100, systolic greater than 140).<br><br>*Procedures*— Ophthalmoscopy: retinopathy, papilledema.<br><br>*Radiology*— Chest x-ray: congestive heart failure; cardiac enlargement. |

| Condition | Documentation |
|---|---|
| **Disorders, papillary muscle** | *Signs and Symptoms:* Sudden development of pulmonary edema. Shortness of breath, edema and severe chest pain. Normally occurs within 10 days of an acute myocardial infarction. Patient usually dies within 24 hours, and 90% die within two weeks.<br><br>*Nurse's Notes*— Frequent monitoring of vital signs and intake and output.<br><br>*Procedures*— Emergency mitral valve or cardiac catheterization using intraaortic balloon pump. Aortocoronary saphenous vein bypass is usually performed. Mitral valve replacement may be performed.<br><br>*Radiology*— Ultrasound of heart or angiography may confirm clinical diagnosis. |
| **Embolism, and infarction, pulmonary** | *Signs and Symptoms:* Manifestations of embolism with infarction include cough, hemoptysis, pleuritic chest pain, fever and signs of pulmonary consolidation of pleural fluid. Indications of an embolism develop abruptly over a period of minutes; those of an infarction over a period of hours. May follow a major surgical procedure after which the patient may have been confined to bed rest.<br><br>*Drug Therapy*— Includes low doses of heparin, analgesics, thrombolytic drugs and dextran administered intravenously.<br><br>*Laboratory*— Arterial blood gas may show poor air exchange. Sputum may show red blood cells. LDH may be elevated.<br><br>*Nurse's Notes*— Checking of pedal pulses, range of motion exercises, encouragement of ambulation and oxygen therapy.<br><br>*Procedures*— Pulmonary arteriography may confirm diagnosis.<br><br>*Radiology*— Chest x-ray: may show pleural effusion or infiltrates. Radioisotope perfusion lung scanning often accompanies ventilation scanning. |

| Condition | Documentation |
|-----------|---------------|
| **Failure, congestive heart** | *Signs and Symptoms:* Dyspnea is present, with orthopnea and paroxysmal nocturnal dyspnea in more advanced failure. Other symptoms include peripheral edema, irritability and weakness. Cyanosis is present on occasion. Heart rate is irregular, and moist rales are present in base of lungs with productive cough. Confusion is usually present. <br><br> *Drug Therapy*— May include digoxin, diuretics and vasodilators. <br><br> *EKG*— Tachycardia and atrial enlargement. <br><br> *Laboratory*— Possible increase in plasma volume above 5 percent of body weight. <br><br> *Nurse's Notes*— Frequent monitoring of vital signs and intake and output, oxygen therapy, bed rest, fluid restriction, daily weights and rotating tourniquets. <br><br> *Procedures*— Echocardiography, cardiac blood pool imaging, pulmonary artery monitoring and cardiac catheterization. <br><br> *Radiology*— Chest x-ray: may show cardiac hypertrophy, pleural effusion or pulmonary venous congestion. |
| **Failure, heart** | *Signs and Symptoms:* Documentation of cardiac insufficiency, fatigue or dyspnea. <br><br> *Radiology*— Chest x-ray: cardiac enlargement. |

| Condition | Documentation |
|---|---|
| **Failure, heart left** | *Signs and Symptoms:* Hypertension, fatigue, cough, frothy sputum, pulmonary edema and dyspnea. Confusion is usually present. Documentation may state that the patient is cyanotic.<br><br>*Drug Therapy*— May include diuretics, digoxin, vasodilators and dobutamine.<br><br>*Laboratory*— Blood gases: oxygen saturation reduced. CO2 tension: less than normal.<br><br>*Nurse's Notes*— Rotation of tourniquets, daily weights, intake and output and frequent vital signs.<br><br>*Procedures*— Pulmonary artery monitoring, pulmonary capillary wedge pressure and echocardiography.<br><br>*Radiology*— Chest x-ray: pulmonary congestion and pleural effusion. |
| **Failure, renal acute** | *Signs and Symptoms:* Lethargy, fatigue, anorexia, nausea, dyspnea, weakness, thirst, oliguria, bradycardia or tachycardia. Can develop as a complication of congestive heart failure, shock or sepsis.<br><br>*EKG*— Arrhythmias of all types due to electrolyte imbalance.<br><br>*Laboratory*— Urinalysis: low specific gravity; high specific gravity if due to prerenal or postrenal factors; RBC; protein; traces of glucose; casts; epithelial cells. Blood: increased WBC during infection; increased BUN and creatinine.<br><br>*Nurse's Notes*— Intake and output, daily weights.<br><br>*Procedures*— Intravenous pyelography, ultrasound of the kidneys and possibly hemodialysis or peritoneal dialysis. |

| Condition | Documentation |
|---|---|
| **Failure, renal, acute, with lesion of renal cortical necrosis** | *Signs and Symptoms:* Lethargy, fatigue, anorexia, nausea, dyspnea, weakness, thirst, oliguria, bradycardia or tachycardia.<br><br>*EKG*— Evidence of arrhythmias (e.g., bradycardia or tachycardia).<br><br>*Laboratory*— Urinalysis: low specific gravity; high specific gravity if due to prerenal or postrenal factors; RBC; protein; traces of glucose; casts; epithelial cells. Blood: increased BUN and creatinine.<br><br>*Nurse's Notes*— Intake and output, daily weights.<br><br>*Radiology*— Kidney x-ray: evidence of cortical necrosis. IVP: clinically diagnostic. |
| **Failure, renal, acute, with lesion of renal medullary (papillary) necrosis** | *Signs and Symptoms:* Lethargy, fatigue, anorexia, dyspnea, weakness, nausea, thirst, oliguria, bradycardia or tachycardia. Seen most commonly in association with conditions such as liver disease and diabetes.<br><br>*EKG*— Evidence of arrhythmias (e.g., bradycardia or tachycardia).<br><br>*Laboratory*— Urinalysis: low specific gravity; high specific gravity if due to prerenal or postrenal factors. Blood: increased RBC, protein, BUN and creatinine.<br><br>*Nurse's Notes*— Intake and output, daily weights.<br><br>*Radiology*— X-ray: may show renal medullary (papillary) lesion. IVP: clinically diagnostic. |

| Condition | Documentation |
|---|---|
| **Failure, renal, acute, with lesion of tubular necrosis** | *Signs and Symptoms:* Lethargy, fatigue, anorexia, nausea, dyspnea, weakness, thirst, bradycardia or tachycardia. Can be associated with other conditions such as shock, sepsis, renal artery surgery and heavy metal poisoning.<br><br>*EKG—* Evidence of arrhythmias (e.g., bradycardia or tachycardia).<br><br>*Laboratory—* Urinalysis: low specific gravity; high specific gravity if due to prerenal or postrenal factors. Blood: increased BUN and creatinine.<br><br>*Nurse's Notes—* Intake and output, daily weights.<br><br>*Radiology—* X-ray: evidence of lesion of tubular necrosis. IVP: clinically diagnostic. |
| **Failure, renal, acute with speci-fied patholog-ical lesion in kidney** | *Signs and Symptoms:* Lethargy, fatigue, anorexia, nausea, dyspnea, weakness, thirst, bradycardia or tachycardia.<br><br>*EKG—* Evidence of arrhythmias (e.g., bradycardia or tachycardia).<br><br>*Laboratory—* Urinalysis: low specific gravity; high specific gravity if due to prerenal or postrenal factors. Blood: increased BUN and creatinine.<br><br>*Nurse's Notes—* Intake and output, daily weights.<br><br>*Radiology—* X-ray: evidence of pathologic lesion in kidney. IVP: clinically diagnostic. |
| **Fibrillation, atrial** | *Signs and Symptoms:* Occurs as a result of other conditions such as congestive heart failure and sepsis or after bypass or valve replacement surgery. Symptoms include palpitations, dyspnea, dizziness, fainting and apprehension.<br><br>*Drug Therapy—* May include digoxin, diuretics and quinidine.<br><br>*EKG—* Atrial rate over 400/minute with a variable ventricular rate. Absence of P waves.<br><br>*Procedures—* Cardioversion and echocardiography. |

| Condition | Documentation |
|---|---|
| **Fibrillation, ventricular** | *Signs and Symptoms:* A life-threatening cardiac emergency. Absence of effective cardiac action resulting in loss of pulse, respirations and blood pressure. Seizures and death can occur.<br><br>*Drug Therapy*— Lidocaine, procainamide, bretylium tosylate.<br><br>*EKG*— Bizarre QRS complexes; ventricular rhythm chaotic and rapid.<br><br>*Nurse's Notes*— Cardiopulmonary resuscitation and oxygen therapy.<br><br>*Procedures*— Cardiopulmonary resuscitation and defibrillation. |
| **Flutter, atrial** | *Signs and Symptoms:* Palpitations, weakness, dizziness, syncope, anxiety and feeling of impending death.<br><br>*Drug Therapy*— May include digoxin, quinidine, propranolol.<br><br>*EKG*— P waves in regular rhythm (250 to 350 per minute). PR interval prolonged, varying with degree of AV block.<br><br>*Nurse's Notes*— Documentation of rapid regular atrial rate between 220 and 360 per minute.<br><br>*Procedures*— Cardioversion, atrial pacemaker and vagal stimulation. |
| **Flutter, ventricular** | *Signs and Symptoms:* Palpitations and dyspnea. Possible transition between ventricular tachycardia and fibrillation.<br><br>*EKG*— Evidence of ventricular flutter, regular rapid rate over 250/minute. |

| Condition | Documentation |
|---|---|
| **Hypotension** | *Signs and Symptoms:* Weakness, fatigue, dizziness, impairment and blurred vision and syncope. Can be caused by a vasovagal response or by drugs that cause orthostatic hypotension such as antihypertensive drugs and antidepressants.<br><br>*Drug Therapy*— Fluid challenge.<br><br>*Nurse's Notes*— Blood pressures taken while patient is lying, sitting and standing. Support hose. |
| **Rupture of chordae tendinae** | *Signs and Symptoms:* Caused by bacterial endocarditis, trauma or sudden compression of thorax. Usually sudden in onset, with pain in the chest. Patient may have dyspnea and weakness.<br><br>*Drug Therapy*— May include use of diuretics for congestive heart failure (e.g., lasix).<br><br>*EKG*— Features of right or left ventricular failure, hypertrophy and axis deviation.<br><br>*Physician's/Nurse's Notes*— Documentation of congestive heart failure.<br><br>*Radiology*— Chest x-ray: cardiac enlargement. |
| **Rupture of papillary muscle** | *Signs and Symptoms:* Contraction of papillary muscle, also ischemia of papillary muscle. Possible chest pain. There is usually sudden and severe deterioration. Possible hemoptysis. Often manifestation of congestive heart failure with cyanosis and sometimes shock. Occurs in 35% of all myocardial infarction patients.<br><br>*Drug Therapy*— May include lasix or diuril.<br><br>*EKG*— Changes in junction J, S-T, T interval, TU segment and U wave.<br><br>*Procedures*— Mitral valve replacement is often performed.<br><br>*Radiology*— Chest x-ray: cardiac enlargement and pulmonary congestion. |

| Condition | Documentation |
|---|---|
| **Shock** | *Signs and Symptoms:* Noted to be failure of peripheral circulation. This category of shock would include shock caused by anaphalaxis, third-degree burns, extensive tissue trauma or general trauma. May be indicated by documentation of respiratory distress, hypotension, tachycardia, cool moist skin and reduced urinary output.<br><br>*EKG*— Tachycardia.<br><br>*Laboratory*— Serum potassium lactate, BUN and specific gravity are increased.<br><br>*Nurse's Notes*— Intravenous blood and fluid replacement, oxygen therapy, frequent monitoring of vital signs, Foley catheter, intake and output and cardiopulmonary resuscitation. |
| **Shock, cardiogenic** | *Signs and Symptoms:* A life-threatening emergency requiring intensive stabilizing measures. Most often occurs as the result of a myocardial infarction, end-stage cardiomyopathy or possibly a malfunction of the mitral valve. Rapidly developing mental confusion with weakness, cyanosis, oliguria, tachycardia and gallop rhythm. Systolic pressure drops to 50. Skin is cool and moist.<br><br>*Drug Therapy*— May include morphine to control chest pain, dopamine, norepinephrine and nitroprusside.<br><br>*EKG*— Ventricular fibrillation may be present.<br><br>*Laboratory*— May show serum acidosis. BUN and creatinine are elevated, as are CPK, LDH, SGOT and SGPT. Arterial blood gases demonstrate acidosis and hypoxia.<br><br>*Nurse's Notes*— May indicate a weak, rapid pulse, cardiac monitoring and intake and output.<br><br>*Procedures*— Pulmonary artery pressure (PAP) monitoring and pulmonary capillary wedge pressure (PCWP). May also include intraaortic balloon pump (IABP).<br><br>*Radiology*— Chest x-ray: may show pulmonary edema. |

| Condition | Documentation |
|---|---|
| **Syndrome, postmyocardial infarction** | *Signs and Symptoms:* Called "Dressler syndrome." Chest pain is usually sharp and stabbing in nature and often as severe as that caused by infarction. Aggravated by change in position and deep inspirations. Usually follows an acute infarction of two to 11 weeks. (Symptoms similar to pleural effusion, pneumonitis with fever.) Pericardial friction rub present on auscultation. |
| | *Drug Therapy—* May include a short intensive course of corticosteroids. Intensive antiinflammatory therapy may be documented. |
| | *Laboratory—* May show increased WBC of 10,000 to 20,000. |
| | *Procedures—* Echocardiography to determine extent of pericardial effusion. Pericardiocentesis may be necessary. |
| | *Radiology—* Chest x-ray: may reveal pericardial and pleural effusion. May show enlargement of silhouette with later reduction or evidence of pulmonary infiltrates. |
| **Tachycardia, paroxysmal** | *Signs and Symptoms:* Fluttering sensation in the chest, weakness, faintness and nausea. |
| | *Drug Therapy—* May include quinidine, procainamide, tambocor disopyramide. |
| | *EKG—* Uninterrupted series of beats. |
| **Tachycardia, parosysmal supraventricular** | *Signs and Symptoms:* Abrupt onset and termination of palpitations. Often asymptomatic, although patient may be aware of a rapid heartbeat. Some patients complain of throbbing vessels of the throat, dyspnea, sweating, dizziness, syncope, weakness and polyuria. |
| | *Drug Therapy—* May include propranolol, quinidine or verapamil. |
| | *EKG—* Premature atrial beats, abnormally shaped P waves, regular rhythm at 150-220 beats per minute. |
| | *Procedures—* May include intracardiac electrophysiologic studies and vagal stimulation. May also see reduced vital capacity and increased cardiac output and circulation time. |

| Condition | Documentation |
|---|---|
| **Tachycardia, paroxysmal ventricular** | *Signs and Symptoms:* Associated with ischemic heart disease, especially myocardial infarction. Precordial pain. Sudden onset usually preceded by premature ventricular beats. Pulse rate of 150-210 beats per minute.<br><br>*Drug Therapy—* May include antiarrhythmic medication (e.g., lidocaine, pronestyl).<br><br>*EKG—* Wide QRS complexes.<br><br>*Nurse's Notes—* Cardiopulmonary resuscitation if pulse is absent. Oxygen therapy.<br><br>*Procedures—* Cardioversion. |

# Chapter 7: Complex Diagnoses

| Condition | Documentation |
|---|---|
| **Angina, chronic, unstable, not otherwise specified** | See Ischemia, coronary and Syndrome, coronary, intermediate |
| **Arrest, cardiac** | *Signs and Symptoms:* Sudden unexpected cessation of cardiac action, absence of heart sounds and/or blood pressure. Loss of consciousness, rapid, shallow breathing. Cardiopulmonary resuscitation performed.<br><br>*Drug Therapy*— May include isoproterenol, atropine, sodium bicarbonate, epinephrine and calcium gluconate.<br><br>*EKG*— Changes prior to arrest may show bradycardia, tachycardia or other arrhythmias, fibrillation, such as ventricular fibrillation, or asystole.<br><br>*Physician's/Nurse's Notes*— Resuscitative efforts recorded in notes or "code sheet."<br><br>*Procedures*— May include intubation and artificial ventilation. May also include defibrillation. |

| Condition | Documentation |
|---|---|
| **Cardiomyop-athy, alco-holic** | *Signs and Symptoms:* Documentation of excessive alcohol intake, exertional dyspnea, cough, fatigue, hemoptysis and edema. This condition is frequently found in patients between 23 and 50 years of age.<br><br>*Drug Therapy*— May include digoxin, pronestyl, diuretics and vasodilators.<br><br>*EKG*— May show atrial enlargement, sinus tachycardia, premature ventricular contractions, atrial fibrillation or ventricular hypertrophy.<br><br>*Nurse's Notes*— Intake and output, daily weights, frequent vital signs and documentation of complete bed rest. Oxygen therapy.<br><br>*Procedures*— Cardiac catheterization, echocardiogram and possible heart transplant.<br><br>*Radiology*— Chest x-ray may show cardiac hypertrophy or pleural effusion. |
| **Cardiomyop-athy, nutri-tional and metabolic** | *Signs and Symptoms:* Underlying disease: thyrotoxicosis, beriberi, amyloidosis. Symptoms include dyspnea, paroxysmal nocturnal dyspnea, fatigue, edema and palpitations.<br><br>*Drug Therapy*— May include digoxin, pronestyl, diuretics and vasodilators.<br><br>*EKG*— May show atrial enlargement, sinus tachycardia, premature ventricular contractions, atrial fibrillation or ventricular hypertrophy.<br><br>*Nurse's Notes*— Intake and output, daily weights, frequent vital signs and documentation of complete bed rest. Oxygen therapy.<br><br>*Procedures*— Cardiac catheterization, echocardiogram and possible heart transplant.<br><br>*Radiology*— Chest x-ray may show cardiac hypertrophy or pleural effusion. |

| Condition | Documentation |
|---|---|
| **Cardiomyopathy, primary** | *Signs and Symptoms:* Usually demonstrated in elderly patients with loss of consciousness, palpitations and/or dyspnea. Palpitations may be evident by bounding or rapid pulse and skipped heart beats. Edema and paroxysmal nocturnal dyspnea also may be present. May include congestive and restrictive cardiomyopathies.<br><br>*Drug Therapy*— May include digoxin, pronestyl, diuretics and vasodilators.<br><br>*EKG*— May show atrial enlargement, sinus tachycardia, premature ventricular contractions, atrial fibrillation or ventricular hypertrophy.<br><br>*Nurse's Notes*— Intake and output, daily weights, frequent vital signs and documentation of complete bed rest. Oxygen therapy.<br><br>*Procedures*— Cardiac catheterization, echocardiogram and possible heart transplant.<br><br>*Radiology*— Chest x-ray may show cardiac hypertrophy or pleural effusion |
| **Cardiomyopathy, secondary** | *Signs and Symptoms:* Hypertrophy of heart. Occurs as a complication of cardiovascular disease or other systemic disease. Symptoms include dyspnea, paroxysmal nocturnal dyspnea, fatigue, edema and palpitations.<br><br>*Drug Therapy*— May include digoxin, pronestyl, diuretics and vasodilators.<br><br>*EKG*— May show atrial enlargement, sinus tachycardia, premature ventricular contractions, atrial fibrillation or ventricular hypertrophy.<br><br>*Nurse's Notes*— Intake and output, daily weights, frequent vital signs and documentation of complete bed rest. Oxygen therapy.<br><br>*Procedures*— Cardiac catheterization, echocardiogram and possible heart transplant.<br><br>*Radiology*— Chest x-ray may show cardiac hypertrophy or pleural effusion. |

| Condition | Documentation |
|---|---|
| **Cardiomyop-athy in other diseases olaooified elsewhere** | *Signs and Symptoms:* Increase in diastolic blood pressure. Loss of consciousness, hypertrophy of heart and/or history of heart disease. Symptoms include dyspnea, paroxysmal nocturnal dyspnoa, fatiguo, odoma and palpitations. Can occur with sarcoidosis, hypertension or muscular dystrophy.
*Drug Therapy*— May include digoxin, pronestyl, diuretics and vasodilators.
*EKG*— May show atrial enlargement, sinus tachycardia, premature ventricular contractions, atrial fibrillation or ventricular hypertrophy.
*Nurse's Notes*— Intake and output, daily weights, frequent vital signs and documentation of complete bed rest. Oxygen therapy.
*Procedures*— Cardiac catheterization, echocardiogram and possible heart transplant.
*Radiology*— Chest x-ray may show cardiac hypertrophy or pleural effusion. |
| **Cardiomyop-athy of Africa, obscure** | *Signs and Symptoms:* Viral in etiology. Destroys heart muscle and tissue. Probable heart failure.
*Drug Therapy*— May include digoxin, pronestyl, diuretics and vasodilators.
*EKG*— May show atrial enlargement, sinus tachycardia, premature ventricular contractions, atrial fibrillation or ventricular hypertrophy.
*Nurse's Notes*— Intake and output, daily weights, frequent vital signs and documentation of complete bed rest. Oxygen therapy.
*Procedures*— Cardiac catheterization, echocardiogram and possible heart transplant.
*Radiology*— Chest x-ray may show cardiac hypertrophy or pleural effusion. |

| Condition | Documentation |
|---|---|
| **Cor pulmonale** | *Signs and Symptoms:* Progressive dyspnea, substernal discomfort or pain, persistent cough, wheezing, fatigue and edema. Documentation of infection. Most commonly results from chronic obstructive pulmonary disease (COPD). |
| | *Drug Therapy—* May include bronchodilators (i.e., alupent, aminophylline, brethine, bronkosol, epinephrine or theophylline) diuretics, vasodilators, digoxin and antibiotics. |
| | *EKG—* Cardiac arrhythmias such as premature atrial and ventricular contractions. |
| | *Laboratory—* Arterial blood gas may show poor air exchange ($pO_2$ 75-100). Hypoxemia is indicated by low $O_2$ saturation ($O_2$ less than 80). Hematocrit is often greater than 50%. |
| | *Nurse's Notes—* Intake and output, daily weights, fluid restriction and low-salt diet. |
| | *Procedures—* Echocardiography or cardiac angiography demonstrating right ventricular hypertrophy. |
| | *Radiology—* Right ventricular hypertrophy and large central pulmonary arteries. |
| | *Respiratory therapy—* May include IPPB treatment, use of $O_2$ in low concentrations for patients with COPD and/or use of bronchodilators. |
| **Defect, cardiac, septal, acquired and other** | *Signs and Symptoms:* $S_2$ sounds normally split in small ventricular defect; soft, early systolic ejection murmur. |
| | *EKG—* P waves normal or peaked. $P_3$ may be inverted in sinus venosus defect. |
| | *Radiology—* Chest x-ray normal or light LVE; little or no increase in pulmonary vasculature in ventricular defects. |

| Condition | Documentation |
|---|---|
| **Disease, hypertensive heart and ronal, bonign, with congestive heart failure** | *Signs and Symptoms:* History of renal disease, headache, fatigue and irritability. History of hypertensive heart disease.<br><br>*Drug Therapy*— Vasodilators such as minoxidil; antihypertensives such as norvasc.<br><br>*EKG*— Possible tachycardia.<br><br>Laboratory:  BUN level greater than 20 and creatinine above 2.5.<br><br>*Nurse's Notes*— Frequent monitoring of vital signs, intake and output and low-sodium diet.<br><br>*Procedures*— Dialysis.<br><br>*Radiology*— IVP may indicate renal disease. |
| **Disease, hypertensive heart and renal, malignant with congestive heart failure** | *Signs and Symptoms:* History of renal disease, headache, fatigue and irritability. Evidence of renal failure. Elevated blood pressure (systolic greater than 160 and diastolic greater than 100).<br><br>*Drug Therapy*— Vasodilators such as minoxidil.<br><br>*EKG*— Possible tachycardia.<br><br>*Laboratory*— BUN level greater than 20 and creatinine above 2.5.<br><br>*Nurse's Notes*— Frequent monitoring of vital signs, intake and output and low-sodium diet.<br><br>*Procedures*— Possible kidney transplant and dialysis.<br><br>*Radiology*— IVP may indicate renal disease. |

| Condition | Documentation |
|---|---|
| **Disease, hypertensive heart and renal, unspecified, with congestive heart failure.** | *Signs and Symptoms:* History of renal disease, headache, fatigue and irritability. History of hypertensive heart disease.<br><br>*Drug Therapy*— Vasodilators such as minoxidil; antihypertensives such as norvasc.<br><br>*EKG*— Possible tachycardia. Laboratory: BUN level greater than 20 and creatinine above 2.5.<br><br>*Nurse's Notes*— Frequent monitoring of vital signs, intake and output and low-sodium diet.<br><br>*Procedures*— Dialysis.<br><br>*Radiology*— IVP may indicate renal disease. |
| **Disease, hypertensive heart, benign, with congestive heart failure** | *Signs and Symptoms:* Elevated blood pressure (systolic greater than 160 and diastolic greater than 100). Symptoms may include headache, fatigue, irritability, dyspnea and cardiac arrhythmia.<br><br>*Drug Therapy*— May include aldomet, apresoline, diazide, lopressor, hydrodiuril, aldactazide or diuril.<br><br>*EKG*— Tachycardia, bradycardia or PVCs.<br><br>*Nurse's Notes*— Frequent monitoring of vital signs, intake and output and oxygen therapy.<br><br>*Procedures*— Ophthalmoscopy: retinopathy.<br><br>*Radiology*— Chest x-ray may indicate cardiac enlargement |

| Condition | Documentation |
|---|---|
| **Disease, hypertensive heart, malignant, with congestive heart failure** | *Signs and Symptoms:* Atherosclerosis, history of uncontrolled blood pressure and history of oliguria with varying degrees of renal insufficiency. Onset of elevated blood pressure is usually sudden in nature.<br><br>*Drug Therapy*— May include diuril, hydrodiuril, reserpine.<br><br>*Laboratory*— BUN greater than 20, creatinine greater than 2.5.<br><br>*Nurse's Notes*— Frequent monitoring of vital signs with evidence of rapidly accelerated high blood pressure (diastolic greater than 100, systolic greater than 140) and sodium-restricted diet.<br><br>*Procedures*— Ophthalmoscopy: retinopathy.<br><br>*Radiology*— Chest x-ray: congestive heart failure. |
| **Disease, hypertensive heart, unspecified as benign or malignant, with congestive heart failure** | *Signs and Symptoms:* Atherosclerosis, obesity, ischemic heart disease, headaches, features of myocardial infarction and paroxysmal nocturnal dyspnea.<br><br>*Drug Therapy*— May include aldactazide, aldomet, inderal, pronestyl, hydrodiuril or lasix.<br><br>*Nurse's Notes*— Frequent monitoring of vital signs with evidence of high blood pressure (diastolic greater than 100, systolic greater than 140).<br><br>*Procedures*— Ophthalmoscopy: retinopathy and papilledema.<br><br>*Radiology*— Chest x-ray: congestive heart failure; cardiac enlargement. |

| Condition | Documentation |
|---|---|
| **Disorders, muscle, papillary** | *Signs and Symptoms:* Sudden development of pulmonary edema. Shortness of breath, edema and severe chest pain. Normally occurs within 10 days of an acute myocardial infarction. Patients usually die within 24 hours and 90% within two weeks.<br><br>*Nurse's Notes*— Frequent monitoring of vital signs, intake and output.<br><br>*Procedures*— Emergency mitral valve or cardiac catheterization using intraaortic balloon pump. Aortocoronary saphenous vein bypass is usually performed. Mitral valve replacement may be performed.<br><br>*Radiology*— Ultrasound of heart or angiography may confirm clinical diagnosis. |
| **Disturbances, heart, functional, following cardiac surgery** | *Signs and Symptoms:* History of cardiac surgery (may have occurred previously or during the present admission). Functional disturbances may be indicated by arrhythmias, level of consciousness, diaphoresis or a drop in blood pressure (diastolic pressure less than 60).<br><br>*Drug Therapy*— May include quinidine, lidocaine or pronestyl.<br><br>*EKG*— Ventricular tachycardia or fibrillation and premature atrial contractions (PACs).<br><br>*Nurse's Notes*— Monitoring of vital signs and dietary restrictions. |

| Condition | Documentation |
|---|---|
| **Embolism and infarction, pulmonary** | *Signs and Symptoms:* Manifestations of embolism with infarction include cough, hemoptysis, pleuritic chest pain, fever and signs of pulmonary consolidation of pleural fluid. Indications of an embolism usually develop abruptly over a period of minutes; those of any infarction over a period of hours. May follow a major surgical procedure after which the patient may have been confined to bed rest. |
| | *Drug Therapy*— Includes low doses of heparin, analgesics, thrombolytic drugs and dextran administered intravenously. |
| | *Laboratory*— Arterial blood gases may show poor air exchange. Sputum may show red blood cells. LDH may be elevated. |
| | *Nurse's Notes*— Checking of pedal pulses, range of motion exercises, encourage ambulation and oxygen therapy. |
| | *Procedures*— Pulmonary arteriography may confirm diagnosis. |
| | *Radiology*— Chest x-ray may show pleural effusion or infiltrates. Radioisotope perfusion lung scanning, often accompanying ventilation scanning. |

| Condition | Documentation |
|---|---|
| **Endocarditis, acute** | *Signs and Symptoms:* Onset of abrupt chills, sweats, weakness, anorexia, malaise, arthralgia and hematuria. Chest pain and possible fever. Painless red-blue lesions on palms or soles and splinter hemorrhages of nail beds. Heart murmur may be present. |
| | *Drug Therapy*— Antibiotic therapy in large doses administered intravenously. |
| | *EKG*— Atrial arrhythmias. |
| | *Laboratory*— Positive blood cultures for 85-95% of patients. Most common pathogens include Streptococcus viridans with subgroups; enterococcus or Streptococcus faecalis; coagulas negative Staphylococci. White blood cell count may be increased or decreased. Erythrocyte sedimentation rate (ESR) is elevated. Urinalysis may show hematuria. |
| | *Nurse's Notes*— Monitoring of intake and output and documentation of bed rest. |
| | *Procedures*— Echocardiogram; surgery may be performed for infection of a cardiac prosthesis or for severe damage to the heart valves. |
| | *Radiology*— Abdominal x-ray: possible spleen enlargement. |

| Condition | Documentation |
|---|---|
| **Endocarditis, bacterial** | *Signs and Symptoms:* Onset is insidious depending upon preexisting damage to the cardiovascular system. Documentation may show malaise, cough, sweating, weakness, history of weight loss and pain in chest, abdomen and extremities. Fever (over 102°). Other indications are skin lesions, increased paresthesia and hematuria. Bacterial endocarditis usually follows rheumatic fever. Heart murmur usually present in subacute endocarditis, but may not be evident in acute endocarditis.<br><br>*Drug Therapy*— Antibiotic therapy in large doses intravenously.<br><br>*EKG*— Atrial arrhythmias.<br><br>*Laboratory*— Positive blood cultures for 85-95% of patients. Most common pathogens include Streptococcus viridans with subgroups; enterococcus or Streptococcus faecalis; coagulas negative Staphylococci. White blood cell count may be increased or decreased. ESR is elevated. Urinalysis may show hematuria.<br><br>*Nurse's Notes*— Monitoring of intake and output and documentation of bed rest.<br><br>*Procedures*— Echocardiogram; surgery may be performed for infection of a cardiac prosthesis or for severe damage to the heart valves.<br><br>*Radiology*— Abdominal x-ray: possible spleen enlargement. |

| Condition | Documentation |
|---|---|
| **Endocarditis in diseases classified elsewhere** | *Signs and Symptoms:* Underlying cause may be documented as blastomycosis (116.0), Q fever (083.0) or typhoid fever (002.0). Excludes bacterial endocarditis. Patient may have arthralgia and possibly purpura. May show elevated temperature (greater than 102°). |
| | *Drug Therapy*— Antibiotic therapy in large doses administrated intravenously. |
| | *EKG*— Atrial arrhythmias. |
| | *Laboratory*— Positive blood cultures for 85-95% of patients. Most common pathogens include Streptococcus viridans with subgroups; enterococcus or Streptococcus faecalis; coagulas negative Staphylococci. White blood cell count may be increased or decreased. ESR rate is elevated. Urinalysis may show hematuria. |
| | *Nurse's Notes*— Monitoring of intake and output and documentation of bed rest. |
| | *Procedures*— Echocardiogram; surgery may be performed for infection of a cardiac prosthesis or for severe damage to the heart valves. |
| | *Radiology*— Abdominal x-ray: possible spleen enlargement. |

| Condition | Documentation |
|---|---|
| **Endocarditis, infective, acute and subacute, in diseases classified elsewhere** | *Signs and Symptoms:* Underlying cause may be documented as blastomycosis (116.0), Q fever (083.0) or typhoid fever (002.0). Excludes bacterial endocarditis. Patient may have arthralgia and possibly purpura. May show elevated temperature (greater than 102°). |
| | *Drug Therapy* Antibiotic therapy in large doses administrated intravenously. |
| | *EKG*— Atrial arrhythmias. |
| | *Laboratory*— Positive blood cultures for 85-95% of patients. Most common pathogens include Streptococcus viridans with subgroups; enterococcus or Streptococcus faecalis; coagulas negative Staphylococci. White blood cell count may be increased or decreased. ESR is elevated. Urinalysis may show hematuria. |
| | *Nurse's Notes*— Monitoring of intake and output and documentation of bed rest. |
| | *Procedures*— Echocardiogram; surgery may be performed for infection of a cardiac prosthesis or for severe damage to the heart valves. |
| | *Radiology*— Abdominal x-ray: possible spleen enlargement. |

| Condition | Documentation |
|---|---|
| **Endocarditis, valve unspecified, unspecified cause** | *Signs and Symptoms:* Incompetence and insufficiency of heart valve. Valvulitis. Nonbacterial thrombotic stenosis of valve. Regurgitation of mitral valve. Inflammatory conditions of heart valve. Symptoms include heart murmur, weakness, intermittent fever, petechiae, arthralgia, and confusion.<br><br>*Drug Therapy*— IV antibiotics.<br><br>*EKG*— May reveal tachycardia.<br><br>*Laboratory*— Blood: anemia (hemoglobin less than 8 and hematocrit less than 28). Urinalysis may show red blood cells. Blood cultures: positive in 85-95% of patients.<br><br>*Nurse's Notes*— Monitoring of intake and output.<br><br>*Procedures*— Echocardiogram may be diagnostic; blood transfusion, surgery for infection of cardiac prosthesis or severe damage to the heart valves.<br><br>*Radiology*— Chest x-ray may show cardiac enlargement. |

| Condition | Documentation |
|---|---|
| **Failure, heart, congestive** | *Signs and Symptoms:* Dyspnea is present with ortho- pnea and paroxysmal nocturnal dyspnea present in more advanced failure. Other symptoms include periph- eral edema, irritability and weakness. Cyanosis is present on occasion. Heart rate is irregular. Moist rales are present in bases of lungs with productive cough. Confusion is usually present.<br><br>*Drug Therapy*— May include digoxin, diuretics, such as lasix, and vasodilators.<br><br>*EKG*— Tachycardia and atrial enlargement.<br><br>*Laboratory*— Possible increase in plasma volume more than 5% of body weight.<br><br>*Nurse's Notes*— Frequent monitoring of vital signs and intake and output, antiembolism hose, low-sodium diet, oxygen therapy, daily weights, fluid restriction and rota- tion of tourniquets.<br><br>*Procedures*— Echocardiography, cardiac blood pool imaging, pulmonary artery monitoring and cardiac cath- eterization.<br><br>*Radiology*— Chest x-ray: may show cardiac hypertro- phy, pleural effusion or pulmonary venous congestion. Kerley B lines may be present. |

| Condition | Documentation |
|---|---|
| **Failure, heart, left and unspecified** | *Signs and Symptoms:* Hypertension, fatigue, cough, frothy sputum, pulmonary edema and dyspnea. Confusion is usually present. Documentation may state that the patient is cyanotic.<br><br>*Drug Therapy*— May include diuretics, digoxin, vasodilators and dobutamine.<br><br>*EKG*— Cardiac hypertrophy and tachycardia.<br><br>*Laboratory*— Arterial blood gases: $O_2$ saturation reduced; $CO_2$ retention: less than normal.<br><br>*Nurse's Notes*— Rotation of tourniquets, daily weights, monitoring of intake and output and frequent vital signs.<br><br>*Procedures*— Pulmonary artery monitoring, pulmonary capillary wedge pressure and echocardiography.<br><br>*Radiology*— Chest x-ray: evidence of pulmonary congestion and pleural effusion. |
| **Fibroelastosis, endocardial** | *Signs and Symptoms:* Cardiac hypertrophy with documentation of peripheral edema. Usually occurs in ages six weeks to six months. In older children, there is usually documentation of poor heart sounds and often tachycardia. In patients over 50, documentation of six to 15 years of heart disease. Possible relationship to mumps virus.<br><br>*EKG*— Left ventricular hypertrophy.<br><br>*Procedures*— Angiocardiography. Fluoroscopy: may be clinically diagnostic.<br><br>*Radiology*— Chest x-ray may show extreme left ventricle enlargement. |

| Condition | Documentation |
|-----------|---------------|
| **Hemoperi- cardium** | *Signs and Symptoms:* Results from a perforating trauma or cardiac rupture after myocardial infarction. Symptoms include precordial pain, substernal oppression and dyspnea. Death can result if emergency measures are not taken immediately.<br><br>*EKG*— May show low to inverted T waves in most leads.<br><br>*Nurse's Notes*— Monitoring of vital signs, intake and output and chest tube care (for patient on whom a thoracotomy was performed).<br><br>*Procedures*— Pulmonary artery catheterization. Aspiration of pericardium. Echocardiography.<br><br>*Radiology*— Chest x-ray may indicate increase in acuity of cardiophrenic angle; shape of heart more globular in recumbent position; widening of the base. |
| **Hyperkinetic heart** | *Signs and Symptoms:* Features of congestive heart failure such as cardiac enlargement, gallop rhythm and tachycardia. Pulse pressure may be elevated (the difference between diastolic and systolic blood pressure is greater than 100).<br><br>*Drug Therapy*— May include lasix.<br><br>*EKG*— Sinus tachycardia.<br><br>*Radiology*— Chest x-ray: cardiac enlargement and increased hilar markings. |

| Condition | Documentation |
|---|---|
| **Ischemia, coronary, acute and subacute** | *Signs and Symptoms:* Arteriosclerotic heart disease, elevated cholesterol, disease of aortic valve, thoracic pain, chest pain with or without exertion, anemia, dizziness, syncope and dyspnea.<br><br>*Drug Therapy*— May include nitroglycerin, lidocaine, pronestyl, digoxin, quinidine and potassium supplement administered intravenously.<br><br>*EKG*— Documentation may indicate subacute ischemia.<br><br>*Laboratory*— Potassium level may decrease, indicating cardiac damage. Enzymes may be slightly elevated. Cholesterol level may be greater than 250. Anemia (hemoglobin less than 8 and hematocrit less than 28) may be present.<br><br>*Nurse's Notes*— May document cardiac monitoring or coronay care unit services.<br><br>*Procedures*— Stress EKG and cardiac catheterization.<br><br>*Radiology*— Echocardiogram, myocardial perfusion studies, gated blood pool imaging. Chest x-ray may show cardiac enlargement and increased hilar markings. |
| **Myocarditis, acute, in diseases classified elsewhere** | *Signs and Symptoms:* Associated with acute pericarditis, influenza and tuberculosis. Precordial and substernal discomfort. Severe dyspnea and pain in the right upper quadrant of abdomen.<br><br>*Drug Therapy*— May include antiarrhythmic drugs to control arrhythmias, antibiotics for underlying infection and antiinflammatory drugs.<br><br>*EKG*— Tachycardia, intraventricular or bundle branch abnormalities.<br><br>*Laboratory*— CPK, SGOT and LDH may be elevated. Viral antibody titers, WBC and ESR are also elevated.<br><br>*Nurse's Notes*— Oxygen therapy, frequent vital signs and documentation of bed rest.<br><br>*Procedures*— Endomyocardial biopsy and echocardiogram.<br><br>*Radiology*— Chest x-ray: cardiac enlargement. |

| Condition | Documentation |
|---|---|
| **Myocarditis, acute, other and unspecified** | *Signs and Symptoms:* May be termed "interstitial." Acute form presents with precordial and substernal discomfort, dyspnea, pain and fever. The predominant physical findings are a friction rub, leukocytosis and rapid sedimentation rate. There may also be evidence of generalized edema and/or ascites. May be complicated by congestive heart failure.<br><br>*Drug Therapy—* May include antiarrhythmic drugs to control arrhythmias, antibiotics for underlying infection and antiinflammatory drugs.<br><br>*EKG—* Tachycardia, intraventricular or bundle branch abnormalities.<br><br>*Laboratory—* CPK, SGOT and LDH may be elevated. Viral antibody titers, WBCs and ESR are also elevated.<br><br>*Nurse's Notes—* Oxygen therapy, frequent vital signs and documentation of bed rest.<br><br>*Procedures—* Endomyocardial biopsy and echocardiogram.<br><br>*Radiology—* Chest x-ray: cardiac enlargement. |
| **Myocarditis, septic** | *Signs and Symptoms:* Viral strains. Influenza viruses. Bacteria.<br><br>*Drug Therapy—* May include antiarrhythmic drugs to control arrhythmias, antibiotics for underlying infection and antiinflammatory drugs.<br><br>*EKG—* Tachycardia, intraventricular or bundle branch abnormalities.<br><br>*Laboratory—* CPK, SGOT and LDH may be elevated. Viral antibody titers, WBCs and ESR are also elevated. Blood culture: positive.<br><br>*Nurse's Notes—* Oxygen therapy, frequent vital signs and documentation of bed rest.<br><br>*Procedures—* Endomyocardial biopsy and echocardiogram.<br><br>*Radiology—* Chest x-ray: cardiac enlargement. |

| Condition | Documentation |
|-----------|---------------|
| **Myocarditis, toxic** | *Signs and Symptoms:* May be caused by one of the following: chemical poisons such as arsenic, excessive doses of drugs or excessive radiation exposure.<br><br>*Drug Therapy*— May include antiarrhythmic drugs to control arrhythmias, antibiotics for underlying infection and antiinflammatory drugs.<br><br>*EKG*— Tachycardia, intraventricular or bundle branch abnormalities.<br><br>*Laboratory*— CPK, SGOT and LDH may be elevated. Viral antibody titers, WBC and ESR are also elevated.<br><br>*Nurse's Notes*— Oxygen therapy, frequent vital signs and documentation of bed rest.<br><br>*Procedures*— Endomyocardial biopsy and echocardiogram.<br><br>*Radiology*— Chest x-ray: cardiac enlargement. |

| Condition | Documentation |
|---|---|
| **Pericarditis, acute, in diseases classified elsewhere** | *Signs and Symptoms:* Often a history of recent respiratory infection. Precordial pain made worse by change of position, swallowing, coughing and deep breathing. Dyspnea, chills and malaise are usually present. Onset is sudden. The underlying condition (e.g., tuberculosis) must also be treated. |
| | *Drug Therapy*— Intravenous antibiotics, corticosteroids and antiinflammatory drugs such as aspirin and indocin. |
| | *EKG*— Tachycardia, S-T segment elevation and atrial arrhythmias. |
| | *Laboratory*— WBCs 15,000-20,000, SGOT increased (above 40 units) and PPD skin test is positive if caused by tuberculosis. Positive gram stain and positive culture. |
| | *Nurse's Notes*— Documentation of complete bed rest, frequent monitoring of vital signs and oxygen therapy. |
| | *Procedures*— Pericardiocentesis: fluid may be hemorrhagic or straw-colored. Echocardiogram if pericardial effusion is present. |
| | *Radiology*— Chest x-ray: usually serial for the purpose of ruling out cause of pleuritic chest pain. May show slight cardiac hypertrophy. |

| Condition | Documentation |
|---|---|
| **Pericarditis, acute, other and unspecified** | *Signs and Symptoms:* Sudden onset of sharp precordial pain, not aggravated by thoracic motion. Chills, fever, weakness and dyspnea.<br><br>*Drug Therapy—* Intravenous antibiotics, corticosteroids and antiinflammatory drugs such as aspirin and indocin.<br><br>*EKG—* Tachycardia, S-T segment elevation and atrial arrhythmias.<br><br>*Laboratory—* WBCs 15,000-20,000, SGOT increased (above 40 units) and PPD skin test is positive if caused by tuberculosis. Positive gram stain and positive culture.<br><br>*Nurse's Notes—* Documentation of complete bed rest, frequent monitoring of vital signs and oxygen therapy.<br><br>*Procedures—* Pericardiocentesis: fluid may be hemorrhagic or straw-colored. Echocardiogram if pericardial effusion is present.<br><br>*Radiology—* Chest x-ray: usually serial for the purpose of ruling out cause of pleuritic chest pain. May show slight cardiac hypertrophy. |
| **Rupture of chordae tendineae** | *Signs and Symptoms:* Caused by bacterial endocarditis, trauma or sudden compression of thorax. Is usually sudden in onset with pain in the chest. Patient may have dyspnea and weakness.<br><br>*Drug Therapy—* May include use of diuretics for congestive heart failure (e.g., lasix).<br><br>*EKG—* Features of right or left ventricular failure, hypertrophy and axis deviation.<br><br>*Nurse's Notes—* Documentation of congestive failure. Daily weights, oxygen therapy, intake and output and frequent vital signs.<br><br>*Radiology—* Chest x-ray: cardiac enlargement. |

| Condition | Documentation |
|---|---|
| **Rupture of papillary muscle** | *Signs and Symptoms:* Contraction of papillary muscle; also ischemia of papillary muscle. Possible chest pain. There is usually sudden and severe deterioration. Possible hemoptysis. Often manifestation of congestive heart failure with cyanosis and sometimes shock. Occurs in 35% of all myocardial infarction patients. |
| | *Drug Therapy*— May include lasix or diuril. |
| | *Nurse's Notes*— Daily weights, frequent vital signs, oxygen therapy and intake and output. |
| | *Procedures*— Mitral valve replacement is often performed. |
| | *Radiology*— Chest x-ray may show cardiac enlargement with pulmonary congestion. |
| **Shock** | *Signs and Symptoms:* Noted to be failure of peripheral circulation. This category of shock would include shock caused by anaphylaxis, third-degree burns, extensive tissue trauma or general trauma. May be indicated by documentation of respiratory distress; hypotension; tachycardia; cool, moist skin; and reduced urinary output. |
| | *Drug Therapy*— Nitrates such as nitroglycerin and isordil. |
| | *EKG*— Tachycardia. |
| | *Laboratory*— Serum potassium, lactate, BUN and specific gravity are increased. |
| | *Nurse's Notes*— Intravenous blood and fluid replacement, oxygen therapy, frequent monitoring of vital signs, Foley catheter and intake and output. Cardiopulmonary resuscitation. |

| Condition | Documentation |
|---|---|
| **Shock, cardiogenic** | *Signs and Symptoms:* A life-threatening emergency requiring intensive stabilizing measures. Most often occurs as the result of a myocardial infarction, end-stage cardiomyopathy or possibly a malfunction of the mitral valve. Rapidly developing mental confusion with weakness, oliguria, tachycardia and gallop rhythm. Systolic pressure drops to <90. Skin is cool and moist, often cyanotic and pale. Pulse may be weak and rapid.<br><br>*Drug Therapy*— May include morphine to control chest pain. Dopamine or norepinephrine administered to reverse hypotension.<br><br>*EKG*— Ventricular fibrillation may be present.<br><br>*Laboratory*— May show serum acidosis. BUN and creatinine are elevated as are CPK, LDH, SGOT and SGPT. Arterial blood gases demonstrate acidosis and hypoxia.<br><br>*Nurse's Notes*— May indicate a weak rapid pulse, cardiac monitoring and intake and output.<br><br>*Procedures*— Pulmonary artery pressure monitoring (PAP) and pulmonary capillary wedge pressure (PCWP). May also include intraaortic balloon pump (IABP).<br><br>*Radiology*— Chest x-ray may show pulmonary edema. |
| **Shock, without mention of trauma** | *Signs and Symptoms:* Onset of abrupt chills, nausea, vomiting and diarrhea. Documentation of extreme exhaustion (prostration), hypotension, fever and chills.<br><br>*Drug Therapy*— Intravenous antibiotics.<br><br>*EKG*— May demonstrate conduction defect and/or ventricular fibrillation.<br><br>*Laboratory*— May show serum acidosis or elevated BUN and creatinine. Positive blood culture.<br><br>*Nurse's notes*— Intravenous fluid administration. Monitoring of intake and output.<br><br>*Radiology*— Chest x-ray may show pulmonary edema. |

| Condition | Documentation |
|---|---|
| **Syndrome, coronary, intermediate** | *Signs and Symptoms:* Patients present with anginal pain. History of chronic coronary insufficiency and possible exacerbation of previous stable angina. "Pending infarction"; also may be called "preinfarction syndrome."<br><br>*EKG*— Cardiac monitoring: usually necessary. S-T segment changes and arrhythmias may be present.<br><br>*Laboratory*— Enzyme studies: normal or not diagnostic.<br><br>*Nurse's Notes*— Usually anginal pain is unrelieved by nitrates and onset of pain is nonexertional.<br><br>*Procedures*— Holter monitor, stress test, percutaneous transluminal angioplasty and bypass surgery.<br><br>*Radiology*— Angiography may show coronary artery disease. |
| **Syndrome, postmyocardial infarction** | *Signs and Symptoms:* Called "Dressler syndrome." Chest pain is usually sharp and stabbing in nature, often as severe as that caused by an infarction. Aggravated by change in position and deep inspirations. Usually follows an acute infarction of two to 11 weeks. Appears like pleural effusion, pneumonitis with fever. Pericardial friction rub present on auscultation.<br><br>*Drug Therapy*— May include a short intensive course of corticosteroids. Intensive antiinflammatory therapy may be documented.<br><br>*Laboratory*— May show increased WBC count of 10,000 to 20,000.<br><br>*Procedures*— Echocardiography to determine extent of pericardial effusion. Pericardiocentesis may be necessary.<br><br>*Radiology*— Chest x-ray may reveal pleural effusion. Also may show enlargement of silhouette with later reduction or evidence of pulmonary infiltrates. |

| Condition | Documentation |
|---|---|
| **Tachycardia, paroxysmal ventricular** | *Signs and Symptoms:* Associated with ischemic heart disease, especially myocardial infarction.  Precordial pain.  Sudden onset usually preceded by premature ventricular beats.  Pulse rate of 150-210 beats per minute. |
| | *Drug Therapy*— May include antiarrhythmic medication, (e.g., lidocaine, pronestyl). |
| | *EKG*— Wide QRS complexes. |
| | *Nurse's Notes*— Cardiopulmonary resuscitation if pulse is absent.  Oxygen therapy. |
| | *Procedures*— Cardioversion. |

# ST. ANTHONY HOSPITAL PRODUCTS ORDER FORM

## 1. SHIP TO: SHIP BOOKS TO ADDRESS BELOW

NAME _____ TITLE _____

FACILITY _____

ADDRESS _____ TELEPHONE _____

CITY _____ STATE ____ ZIP ____ FAX _____

## 2. ORDER INFORMATION

| Qty. | Product | Code | Price | Total |
|------|---------|------|-------|-------|
| **1998 ICD-9-CM CODE BOOKS** | | | | |
| ____ | Softbound, Illustrated ICD-9-CM Code Book | SIAS | $ 99.95 | $ ____ |
| ____ | Illustrated, Updatable ICD-9-CM Code Book With Full Text Refill in October | IAD | $ 199.00 | $ ____ |
| ____ | Softbound, Color Coded ICD-9-CM Code Book | CCS | $ 74.95 | $ ____ |
| ____ | Color Coded, Updatable ICD-9-CM Code Book With Full Text Refill in October | ICD | $ 149.00 | $ ____ |
| ____ | Color Coded ICD-9-CM Code Book for Outpatient Services With Full Text Refill in October | OUT | $ 159.00 | $ ____ |
| **1998 APG and GROUPER RESOURCES** | | | | |
| ____ | APG Implementation Guide | AOPR | $ 249.00 | $ ____ |
| ____ | APG SourceBook | APRM | $ 199.00 | $ ____ |
| ____ | APG GuideBook | APG | $ 79.00 | $ ____ |
| ____ | DRG Guidebook | DRG | $ 79.95 | $ ____ |
| ____ | DRG Optimizer | OPT | $ 149.00 | $ ____ |
| ____ | ASC Guidebook | ASC | $ 199.00 | $ ____ |
| ____ | APG Report (newsletter) [ ] 1 yr (12 issues) $249  [ ] 2 yr $448  [ ] 3 yr $596 | APN | | $ ____ |
| **NEWSLETTERS** | | | | |
| ____ | Clinical Coding for Reimbursement [ ] 1 yr (12 issues) $169  [ ] 2 yr $304  [ ] 3 yr $406 | CFR | | $ ____ |
| ____ | HCPCS Report [ ] 1 yr (12 issues) $269  [ ] 2 yr $484  [ ] 3 yr $646 | HCP | | $ ____ |
| ____ | Uniform Billing and Payment Report [ ] 1 yr (12 issues) $269  [ ] 2 yr $484  [ ] 3 yr $646 | FPP | | $ ____ |

## 3. PAYMENT METHOD

[ ] Bill me (add $5.00 Invoicing fee)

[ ] Check Enclosed    [ ] Invoice P.O.#

Make Checks payable to: St. Anthony Publishing
Mail to: P.O. Box 96561 • Washington, D.C. 20090

[ ] Credit Card: [ ] Visa    [ ] MasterCard    [ ] Amex

CA, OH and VA Residents Add Sales Tax $ ____

Invoicing fee $ ____

S & H $ 7.95

TOTAL $ ____

ACCT # _____  EXP DATE _____

SIGNATURE _____

**100% Money Back Guarantee**
If for any reason you are not completely satisfied, return
your purchase within 30 days for an exchange or full refund.

**For fastest service call toll-free 1-800-632-0123 and mention priority code 9296, or Fax (703) 707-5700**